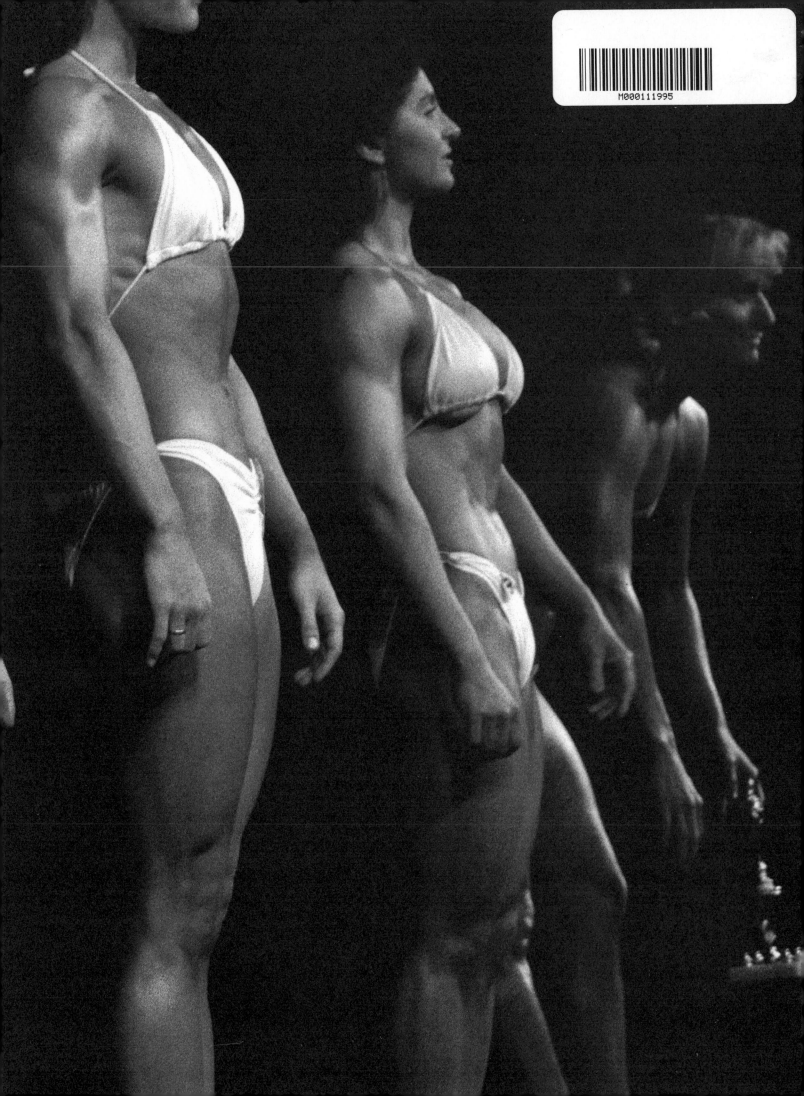

BODYBUILDING
FOR WOMEN

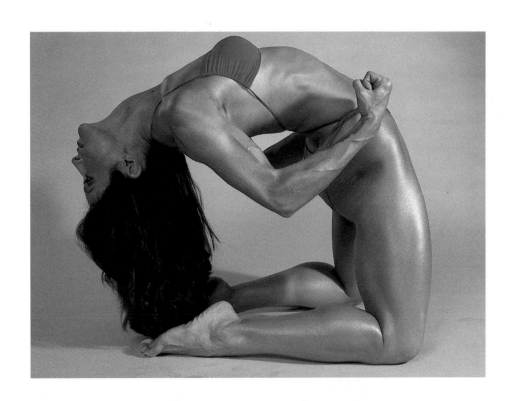

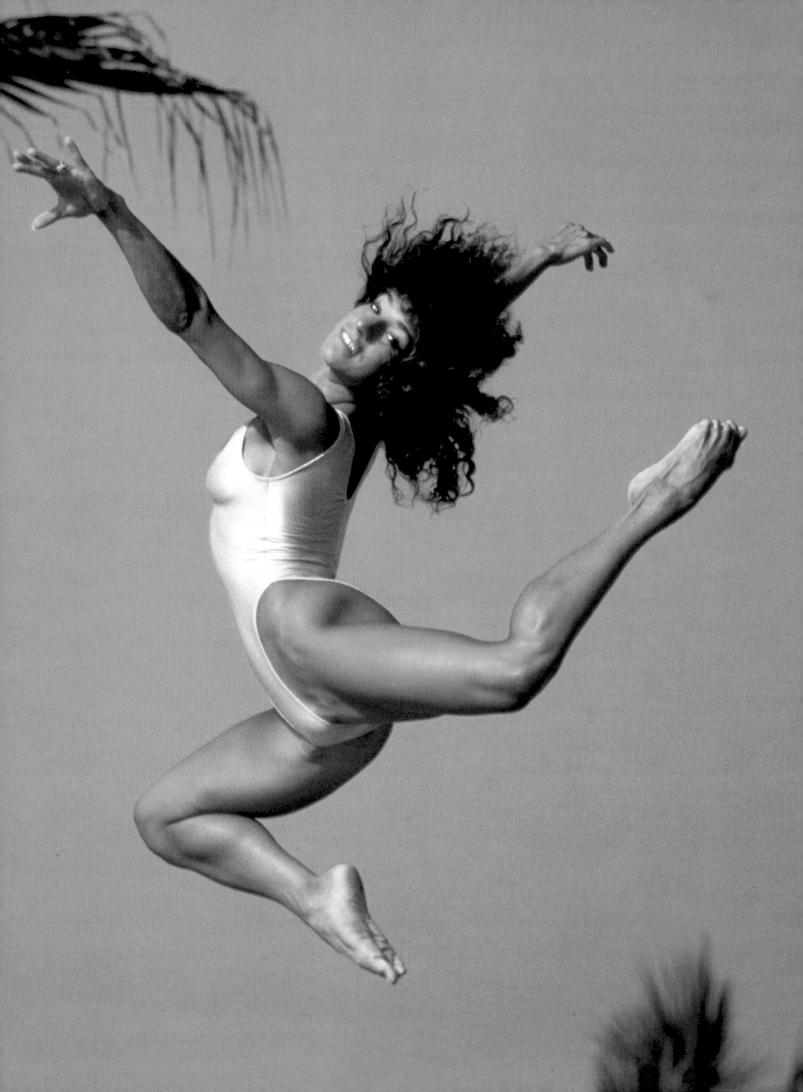

BODYBUILDING FOR WOMEN

OSCAR HEIDENSTAM

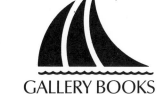

GALLERY BOOKS
An Imprint of W. H. Smith Publishers Inc.
112 Madison Avenue
New York City 10016

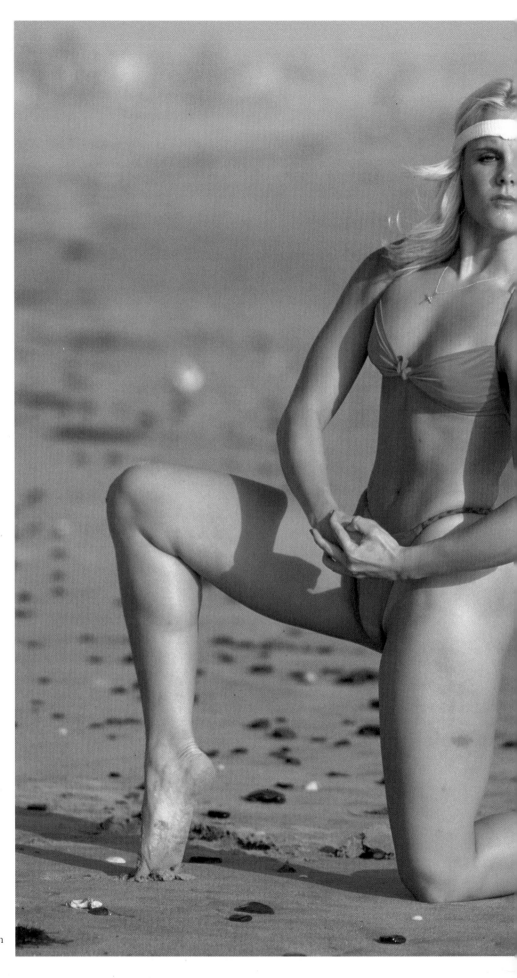

All the exercises in Section II were photographed at The Club On The Park, *London, and the author and publisher would like to thank* The Club On The Park *for all their help.*

The photographs in Section II are by Chris Sowe *and the exercises demonstrated by* Jackie Foster *and* Wendy Page.

This book was devised and produced by Multimedia Publications (UK) Ltd

Editor: Jeff Groman
Production: Arnon Orbach
Design: Terry Allen
Picture Research: Mick Alexander

First published in the United States of America 1985 by Gallery Books, an imprint of W. H. Smith Publishers Inc., 112 Madison Avenue, New York, NY 10016.

ISBN 0 8317 0929 4

Typeset by Keene Graphics Ltd, London
Origination by D S Colour International Ltd, London
Printed in Italy by Sagdos

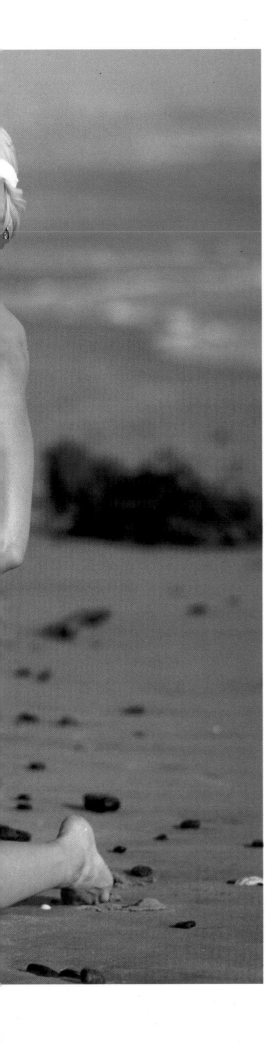

CONTENTS

INTRODUCTION: HEALTH IS PRECIOUS

Section I of this book is a general introduction to the practice of bodybuilding. Section II constitutes a step-by-step guide in color to all the basic exercises described in Section I.

Modern life is tough and complex. It makes great demands on our physical and mental stamina. Accidents will always happen, and no matter how careful we are, serious illnesses cannot always be avoided. But if we keep fit we will be less accident-prone and infection will find it harder to break through our defenses. Let yourself drop below par and you fall an easy victim to disease. You catch every cold easily, and vague headaches, backaches and nervous troubles are always interfering with your everyday life.

You just cannot afford to go on being only half alive. You may have a career before you, or you may have a house to run and children to bring up. Like so many women today, you may be coping with both a career and a home.

There is no doubt about it. A woman must be really fit to keep up with the pace of modern life, and only when she is fit will she realize how much it means. Fitness is not such a difficult goal, if you will take the trouble to learn something about your body and how to keep it in perfect working order with the minimum of effort.

Yet so very many women can't, or won't, bother. They sadly resign themselves to middle age when hardly out of their twenties. They have two children and let themselves go. They suffer bad teeth, poor complexions, varicose veins, aching feet, postural defects, and all sorts of minor ailments. They just don't know how to take care of their bodies.

It's strange, isn't it? Women are traditionally more conscious of their looks and figures than men, yet men have been much quicker to realize the benefits of regular exercise — such as bodybuilding — to keep their bodies looking and feeling good.

I must repeat this over and over again, because it is so very important. Cosmetics and pills cannot restore your looks, retard premature old age, bring back supple curves and that youthful sparkle into your eyes. Only good health can do that, and good health can only be achieved through fitness.

Your body is a machine, and all machines need regular attention. Yet a woman will abuse her body and ignore all the elementary rules of maintenance. Then she wonders why her looks suffer. She wonders why she is beginning to look older than her years.

Here are the 'seven deadly sins' that lead to premature aging.

Faulty diet

There's no need to fuss about diet. But try and cut down on those odd cups of tea with sugar. Don't make do with coffee and a cigarette when you should be eating a square meal.

Lack of exercise

You jump into the car daily, take a walk in the park occasionally when it's fine, swim only when on holiday. It's not enough. Household chores are not sufficient either. You need carefully designed exercise.

Poor personal hygiene

Of course you should take plenty of baths and clean your teeth at least twice a day. And no matter how late to bed you are after a special evening, always remove all make-up and wash your face and neck before going to bed.

Lack of sleep

Late nights once in a while are fine, but don't make a habit of it. Your body needs sound sleep to restore itself. Sound sleep, without the aid of sedatives, only comes with good health.

Faulty posture

Many jobs create postural defects, and nothing shows your age more than the way you stand and walk. Exercises can do a lot for posture. Don't wear tight shoes. And try not to wear shoes with too high a heel. Remember, aching feet show in your face.

Negative mental outlook

A woman is as old as she feels — never forget that. If you are fit and in good health you will feel young and you will look young.

Bad habits

It is easier to start smoking and drinking than to stop. If you haven't yet started, don't. If you have, cut down and do your best to cut it out.

If you want to be fit and healthy and to enjoy life to the full, then you can make a useful start by turning the 'seven deadly sins' into 'seven healthgiving virtues'. How do you achieve this? By spending just 45 minutes three times a week in the invigorating pursuit of bodybuilding.

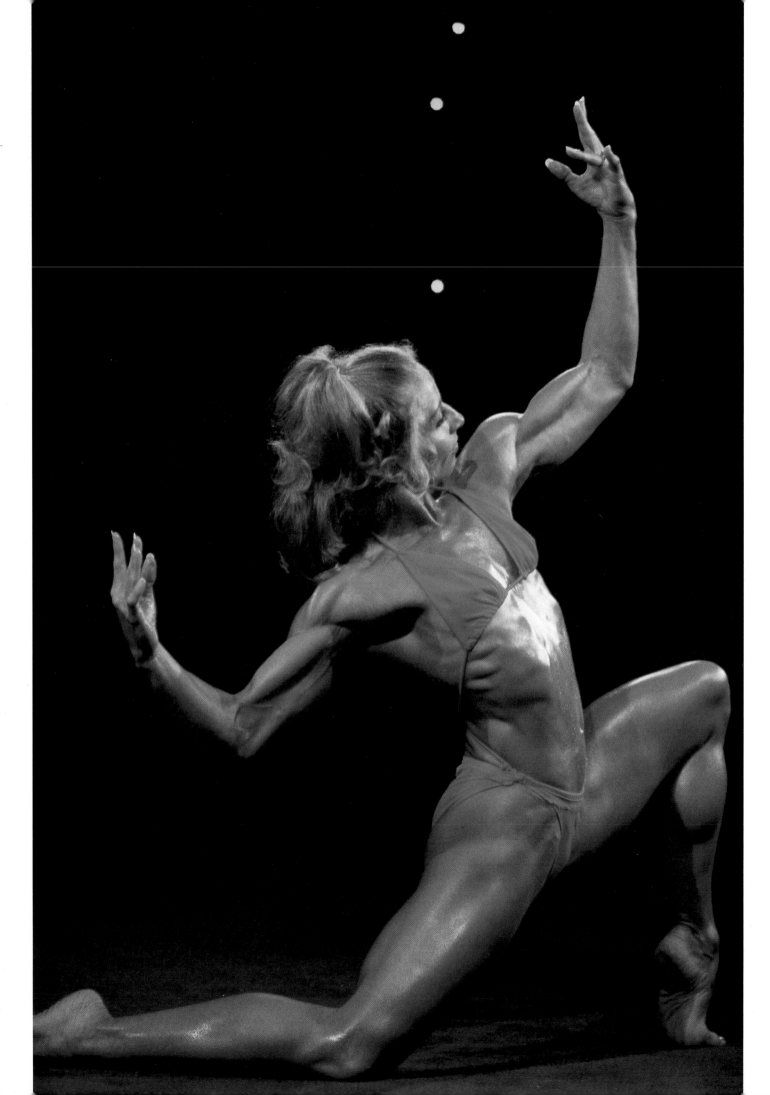

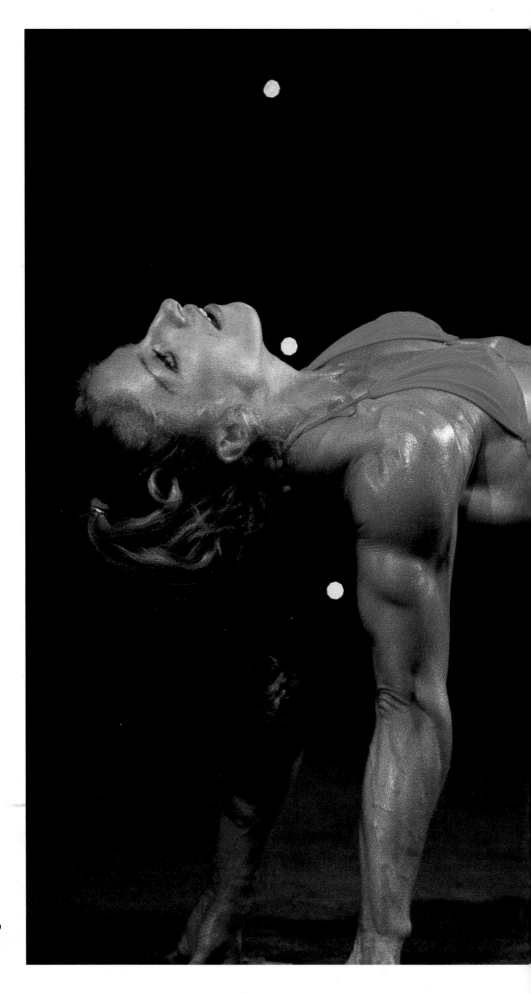

Right and previous page *Kay Baxter of the USA demonstrating the suppleness and agility that bodybuilding brings.*

Following pages *One of the USA's top bodybuilders — Rachel McLish, and one of the most glamorous.*

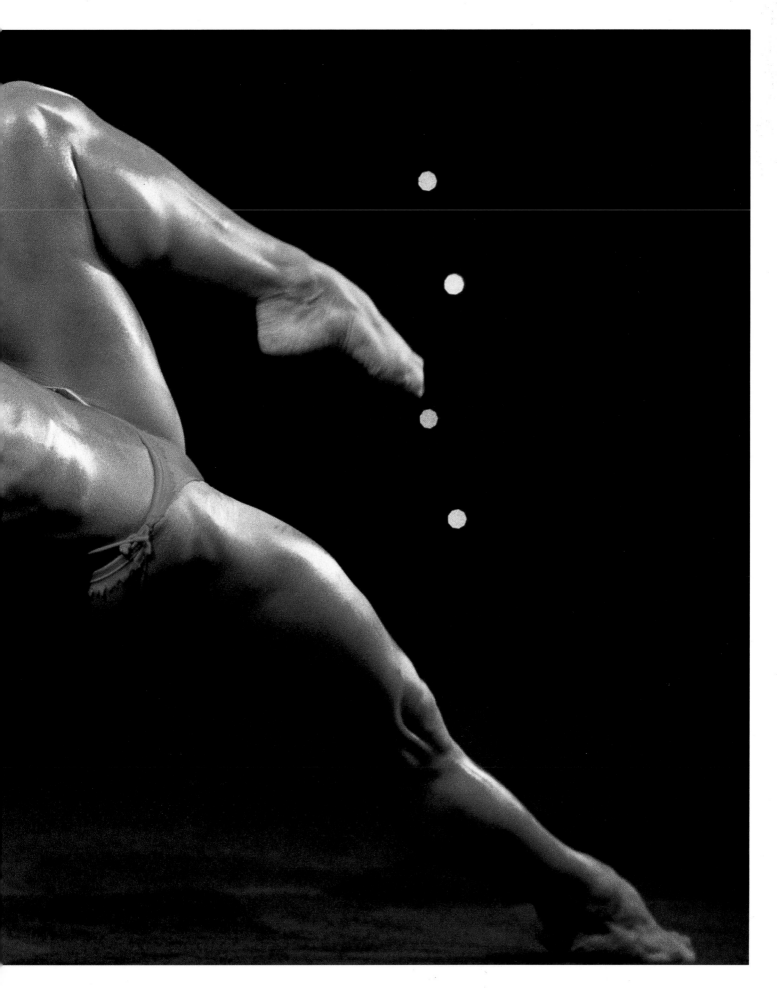

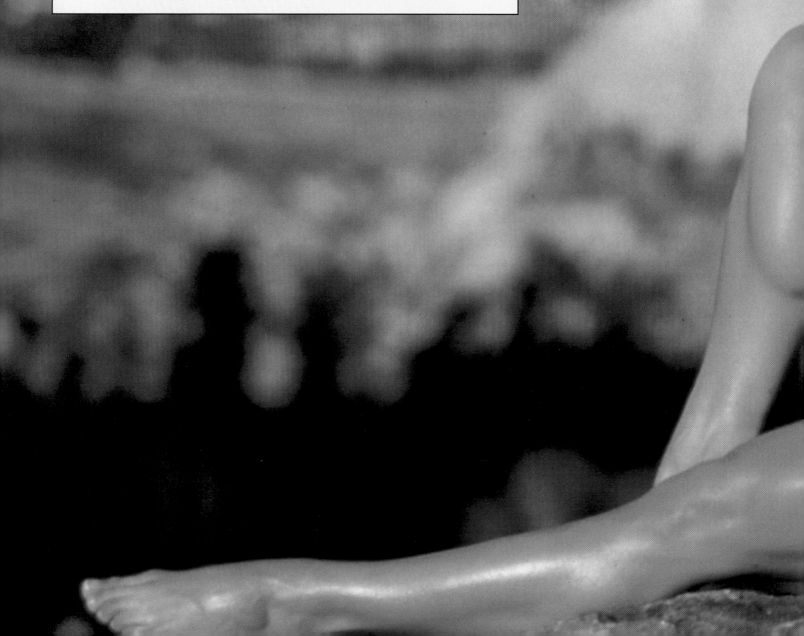

SECTION I:
THE BASICS OF BODYBUILDING

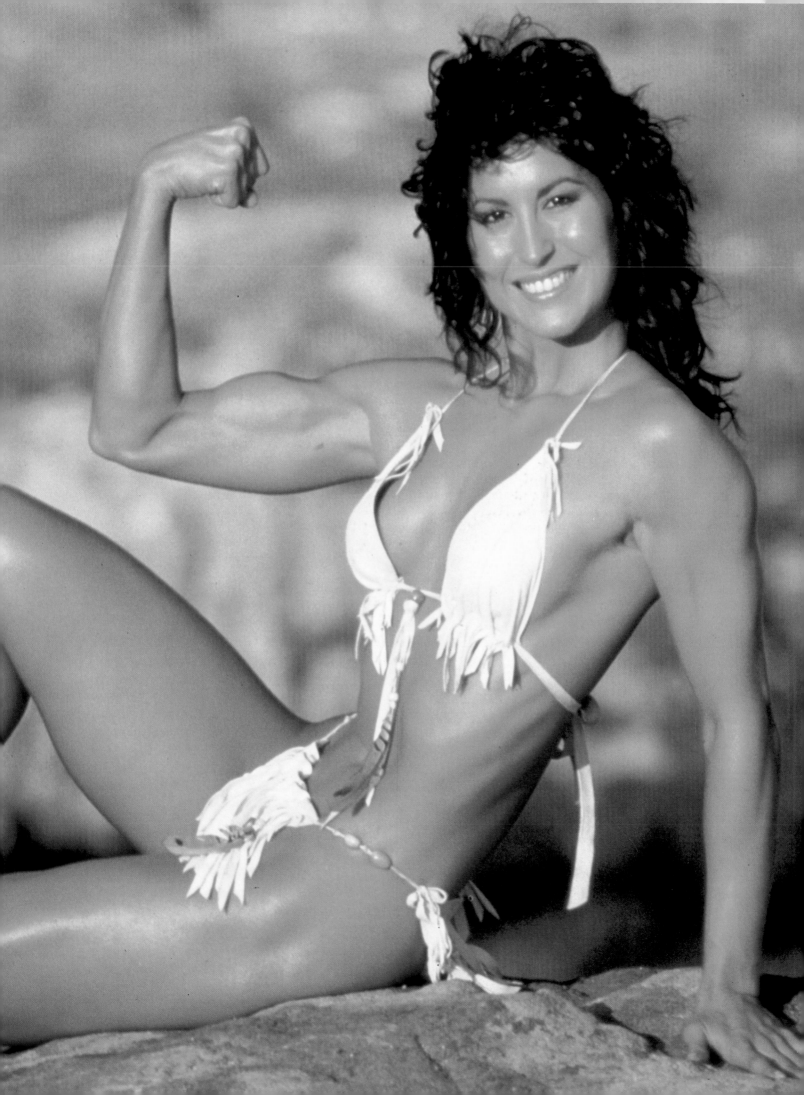

WOMEN AND FITNESS

Bodybuilding exercises for women are not entirely new. Some women were doing weight-training, or resistance exercises, many years ago, but in a very light and cautious way. As with their male counterparts, there were the circus queens and strongwomen acts. But however great their feats of strength, these women were generally looked upon with some suspicion as being rather masculine.

Many women still ask if bodybuilding exercises will make them muscular. The answer is 'not visibly', unless, like their male counterparts, they use specialized training techniques to do so. Even then, women will never develop the same volume of muscle as men bodybuilders.

Today we talk about 'sportspeople' rather than 'sportsmen' or 'sportswomen'. This is because in recent years we have seen that in all sports women are capable of almost incredible feats of endurance and strength. At many events women are breaking records which some 40 years ago were world marks set by men.

In this age of sex equality, women are no longer afraid to attempt any type of sport or exercise which before was almost exclusively reserved for men.

For a long time now, women athletes — like men — have been doing bodybuilding exercises to help them improve their performances. Now women in all walks of life, and of all age groups, have discovered that bodybuilding exercises can be used to promote all-round figure improvement and health. Also these exercises go a long way to help them retain their youth and beauty.

Bodybuilding, if correctly planned, can reduce or add weight, and add or take away inches. You can also concentrate on any specific area of your body, because there is so much scope within the exercises. In this it differs from other sports, which will no doubt keep you fit and healthy, but will not improve any particular aspect of your figure.

Aerobics is a recent trend, and like all forms of exercise is enjoyable — but it has its limitations. Often women, whether they are beginners, young or old, are plunged in at the deep end by joining an aerobics class in which there are not enough instructors to break them up into small groups according to their ability. As a result, beginners are mixed in with more advanced pupils. Bodybuilding, on the other hand, can be planned to suit your own ability by grading the poundages, with repetitions planned to suit you. And there's no need to be part of an embarrassingly overlarge class.

Jogging is very popular for women, but this, too, has had a mixed reception from the experts. How far and how often should you run? Jogging no doubt strengthens the cardiovascular system (heart), but it can be risky with the temptation to jog too far. And jogging on hard roads often plays havoc with your feet and ankles. Bodybuilding can give you all the benefits of jogging — but with none of the drawbacks or hidden dangers.

Approach bodybuilding with confidence, and you will soon discover that as an all-round system for achieving health, fitness and an enviable figure — whatever your age or body type — there is nothing else quite like it. Bodybuilding will make you look more feminine, it will make you move faster on your feet, you will become firmer and less prone to minor injuries — and it may even improve your sex life!

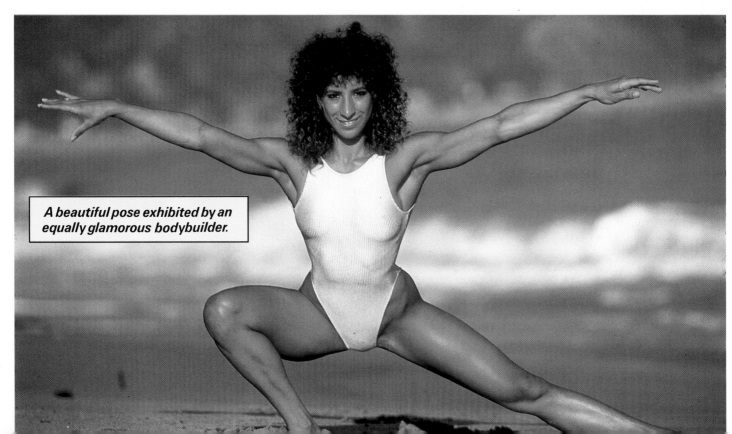

A beautiful pose exhibited by an equally glamorous bodybuilder.

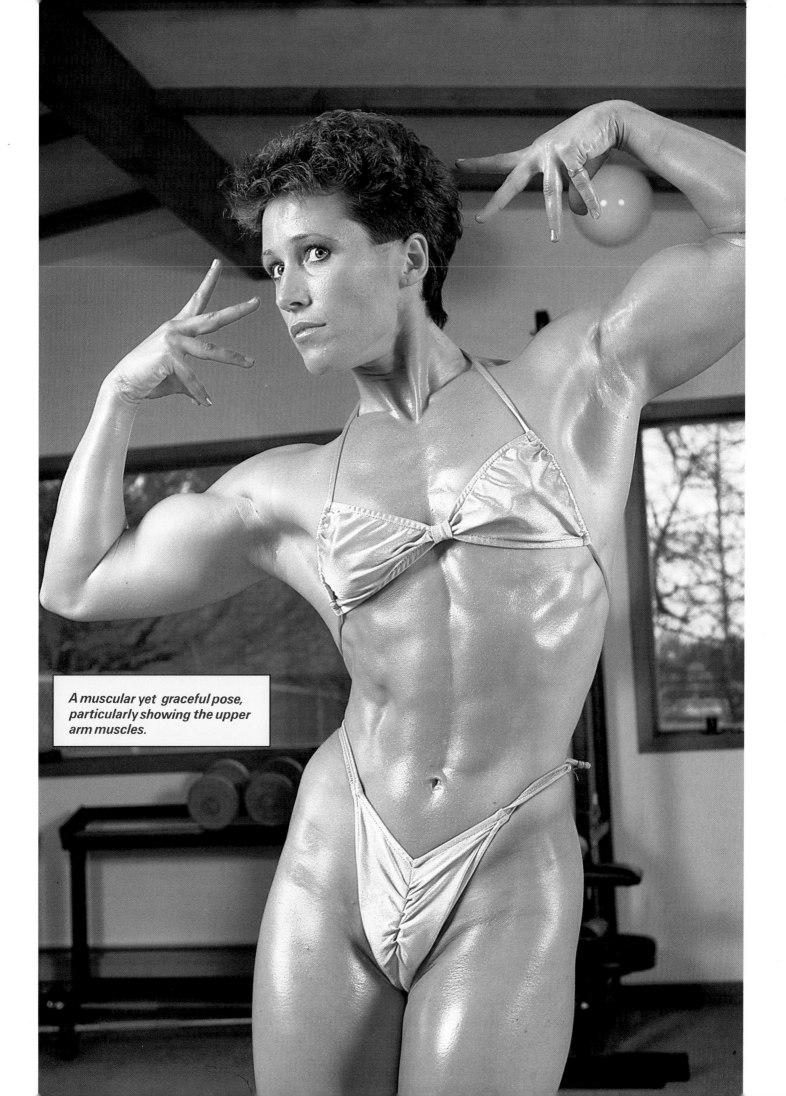

A muscular yet graceful pose, particularly showing the upper arm muscles.

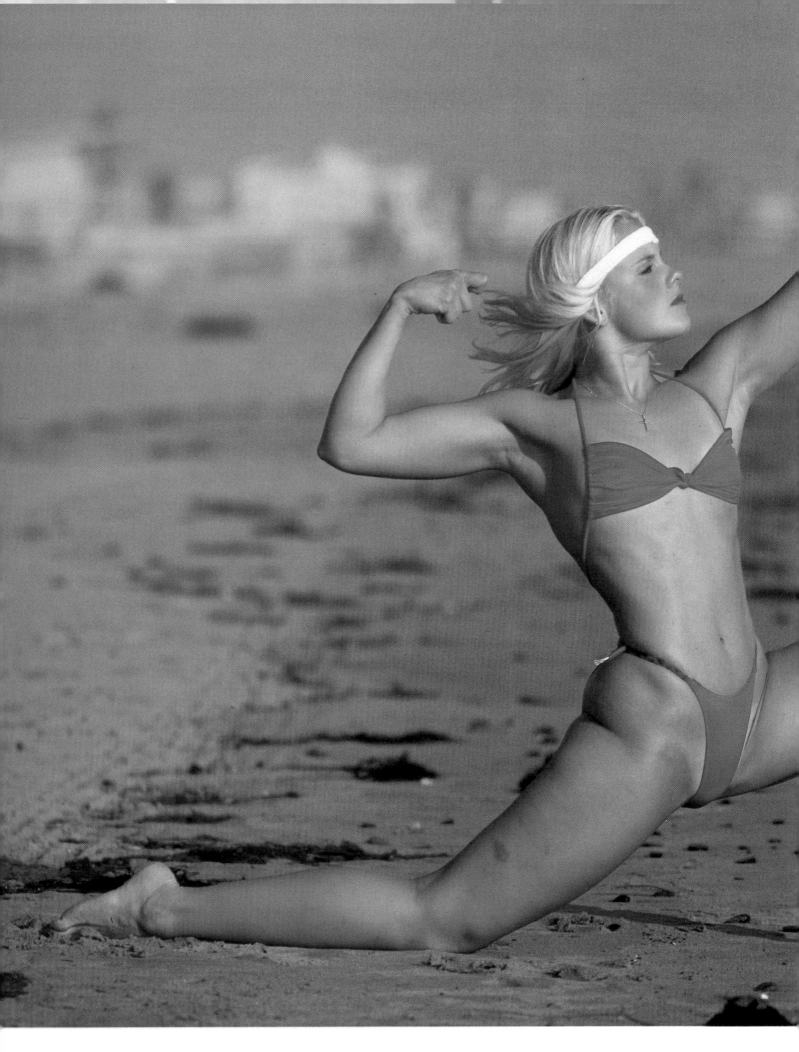

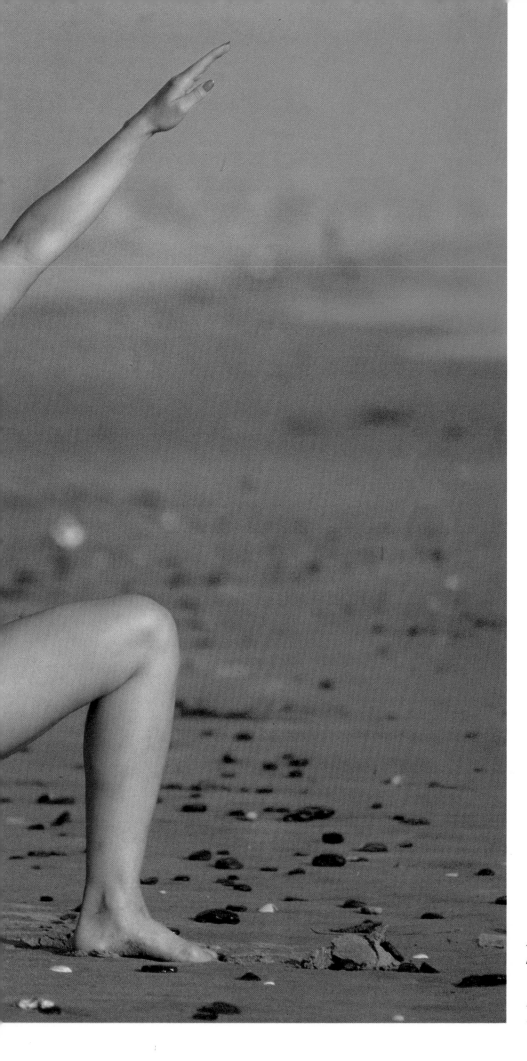

A young bodybuilder posing at the peak of her form. Whatever your body type, a regular bodybuilding workout will guarantee longlasting improvements in your body shape, fitness and wellbeing.

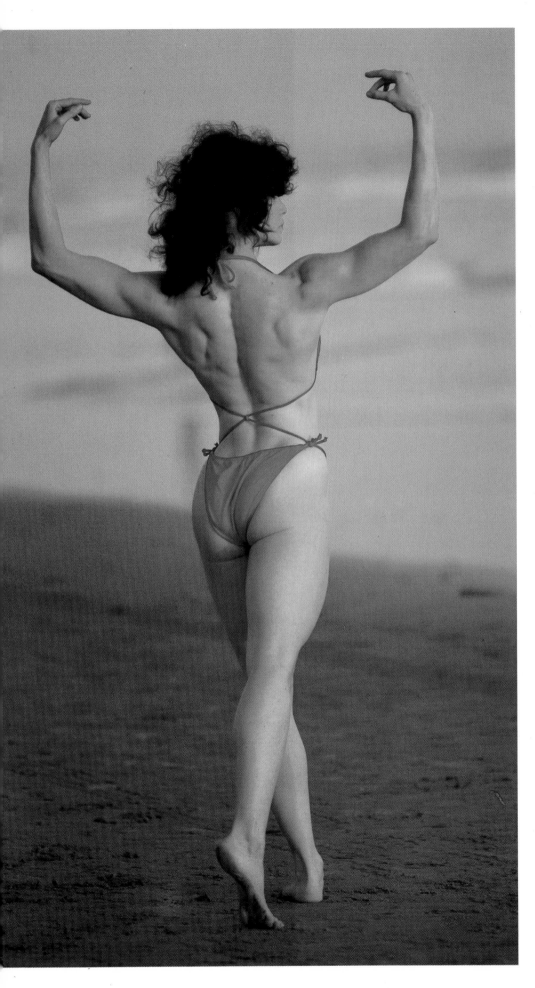

Left *Grace and suppleness are both needed for this bodybuilding pose.*

Right *Liz Karp of the USA shows off her sensational physique — the result of dedicated bodybuilding — helped by a superbright smile!*

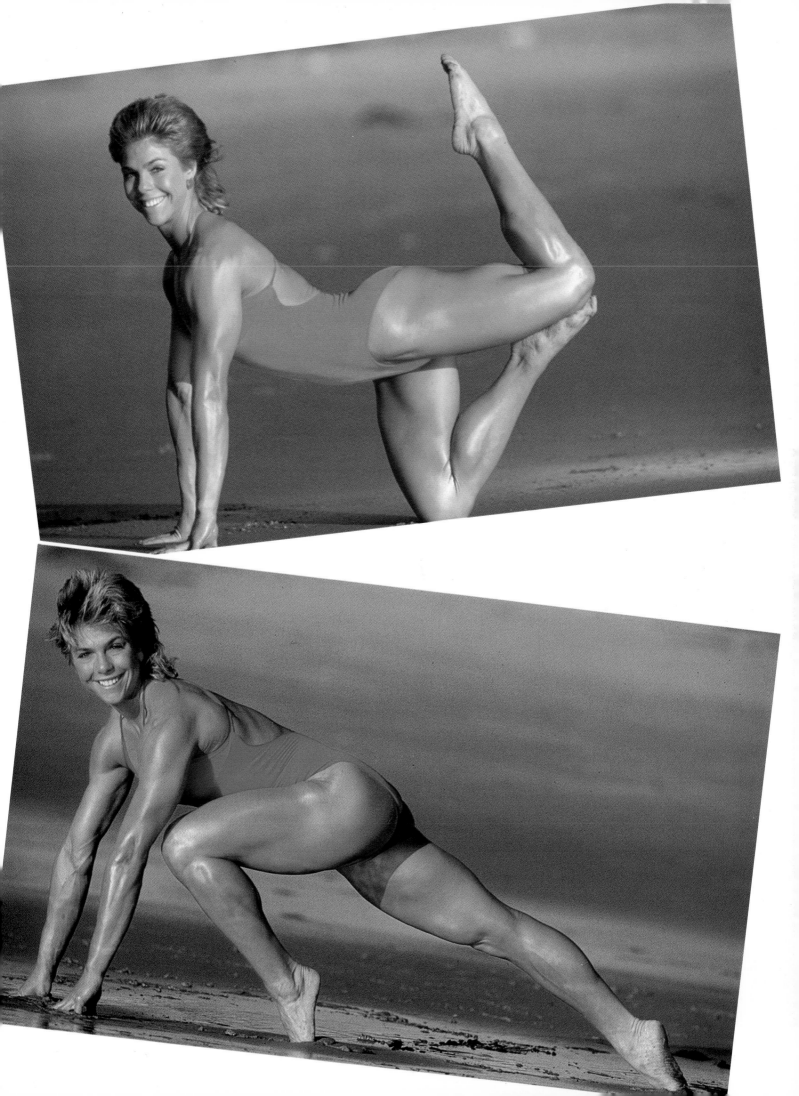

YOUR VITAL STATISTICS

Your weight varies greatly with your body type. And getting to know something of your physical type will save you from disappointment and dissuade you from trying to achieve the impossible through bodybuilding.

A person's physical type is entirely dependent on his or her bone structure. A quick guide can generally be provided by the size of your wrists and ankles, because there is usually very little flesh there, and also by the formation of your rib cage. In both men and women, you will notice that the angle formed by the two sets of ribs coming away from the breastbone may be narrow, or it may almost form a complete semicircle.

The three main body types are: *ectomorph*, or light-boned; *mesomorph*, medium-boned; and *endomorph*, big-boned. Many people are a mixture of more than one type. Some women, for example, may have a light narrow top, and thick, heavy legs, whereas some very heavy women have quite spindly legs.

If you look at some of the statues in a museum or an art gallery, you will see that Aphrodite, the goddess of love, was the small-boned, rather fragile type — a typical ectomorph. Diana, the huntress, was the slender, athletic type, and therefore a mesomorph. The famous Venus de Milo, for so many years idolized for her beautiful figure, was the typical endomorph, with her large hips and quite modest bust.

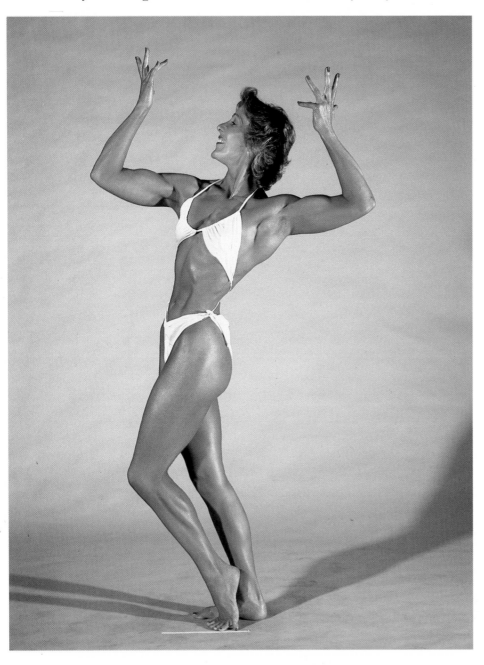

Left *Top international Beth Lopez of Australia has won many titles.*

Right *Vivacious and glamorous bodybuilder Gladys Portugues of the USA. A great deal of hard training has gone into this young lady's physique.*

18

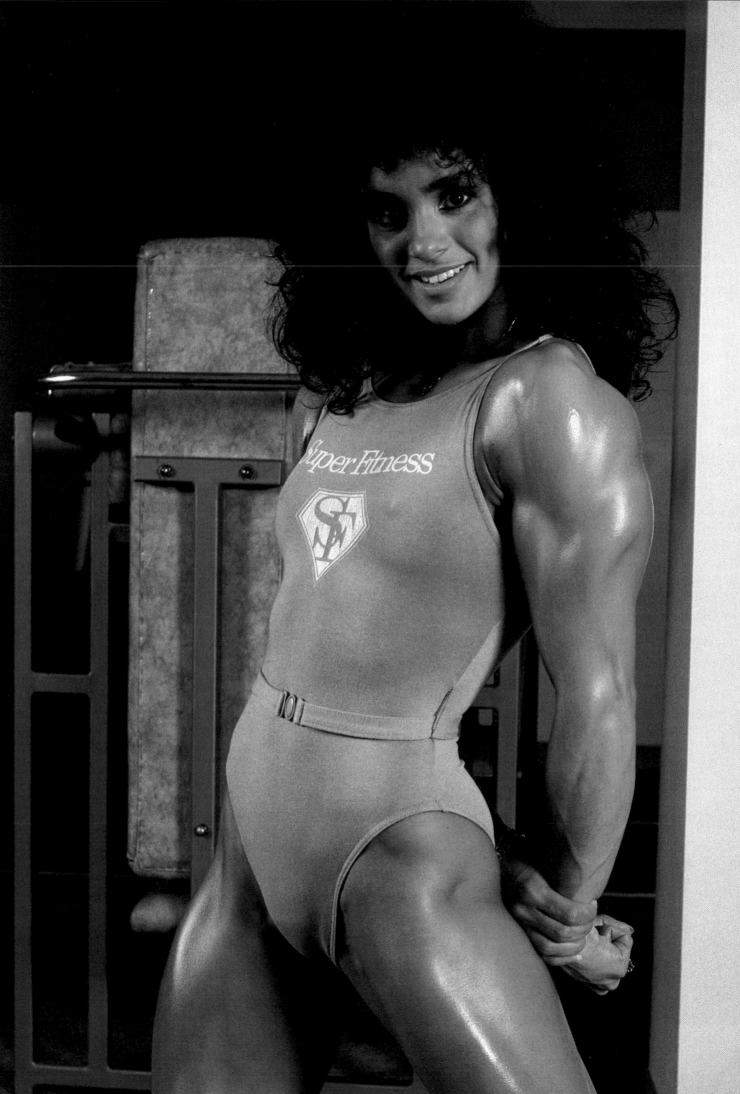

Experts can virtually tell you which sport or event you will succeed at by assessing your physical type. Of course, your type will depend on ancestry, family history, and even what part of the world you come from. In general, the Japanese are small and light boned, whereas Scandinavians, for example, are probably much heavier types.

Ectomorphs have a very narrow angle to their rib cage. They are usually slow gainers and do not put on weight as readily as the other types. They have small wrists and ankles.

Most top athletes and sportswomen belong to the mesomorph type, and the angle of their ribs is wider than that of the ectomorphs. Their wrists and ankles are average in size. Endomorphs have almost a semicircle angle in their rib cages and their wrists and ankles are bigger.

Generally speaking, the light-boned woman has a bust measurement slightly smaller than her hips, which may be wide compared to the rest of her measurements. She is often highly strung, and possibly shy. She finds it hard to gain weight, and can therefore generally eat what she likes. But this does not mean that a correct diet will not improve her health enormously.

The medium-boned woman is physically the athletic type, although she may not want to indulge in any sport. But if she does, she is more likely to succeed. She usually has long legs, a small waist, and a smaller hip measurement than her bust. Normally placid, she mixes well with both men and women.

The endomorph is the heavy-boned woman, often with a large bust. She is not energetic and gains weight easily,

even if her eating habits are modest. A strict diet is a necessity if she wants to keep moderately slim.

From the above, you can get some idea of what body type you belong to. If you really want to improve your figure and your health, you may find it easier to stick to a program if you are of the mesomorphic type (medium-boned), than if you belong to either of the other two.

It's probably true to say that the mesomorphic (medium-boned) type of woman will make the most rapid improvements in appearance after starting a bodybuilding course. However, whatever your body type, bodybuilding exercises — if performed regularly and properly — will *guarantee* improvements in your general body shape, fitness, and wellbeing.

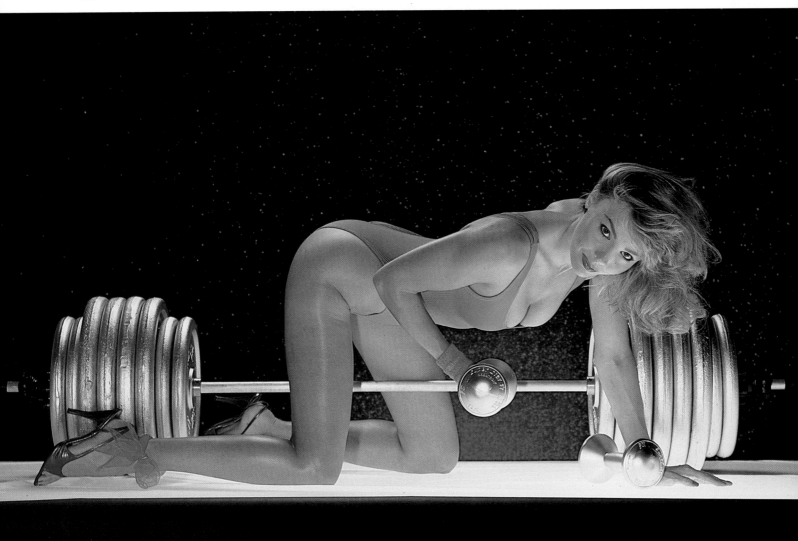

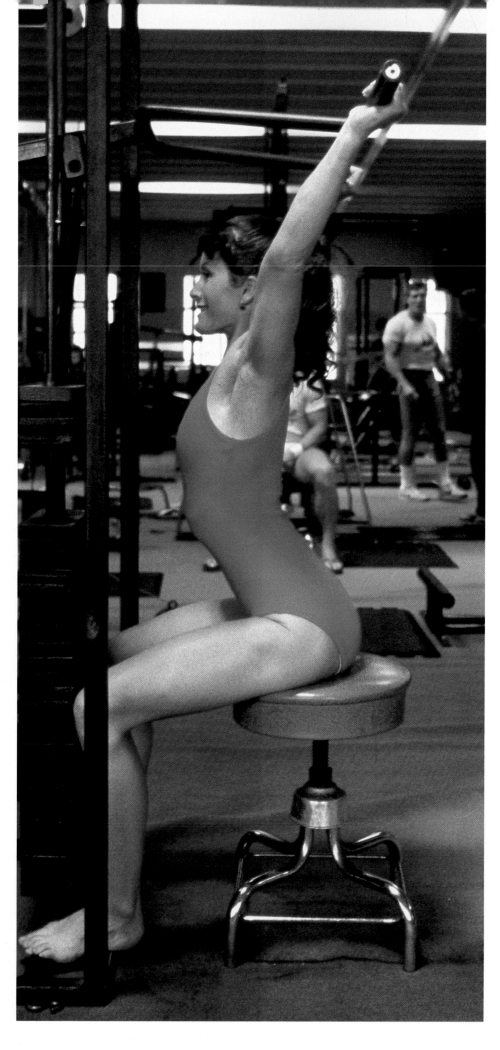

Far left *If you want to achieve — and keep — a figure like this, then bodybuilding is definitely the answer. But you won't need all these weights!*

Left *Performing a pulley pull to the back of the neck — good for the upper back, shoulders and arms.*

21

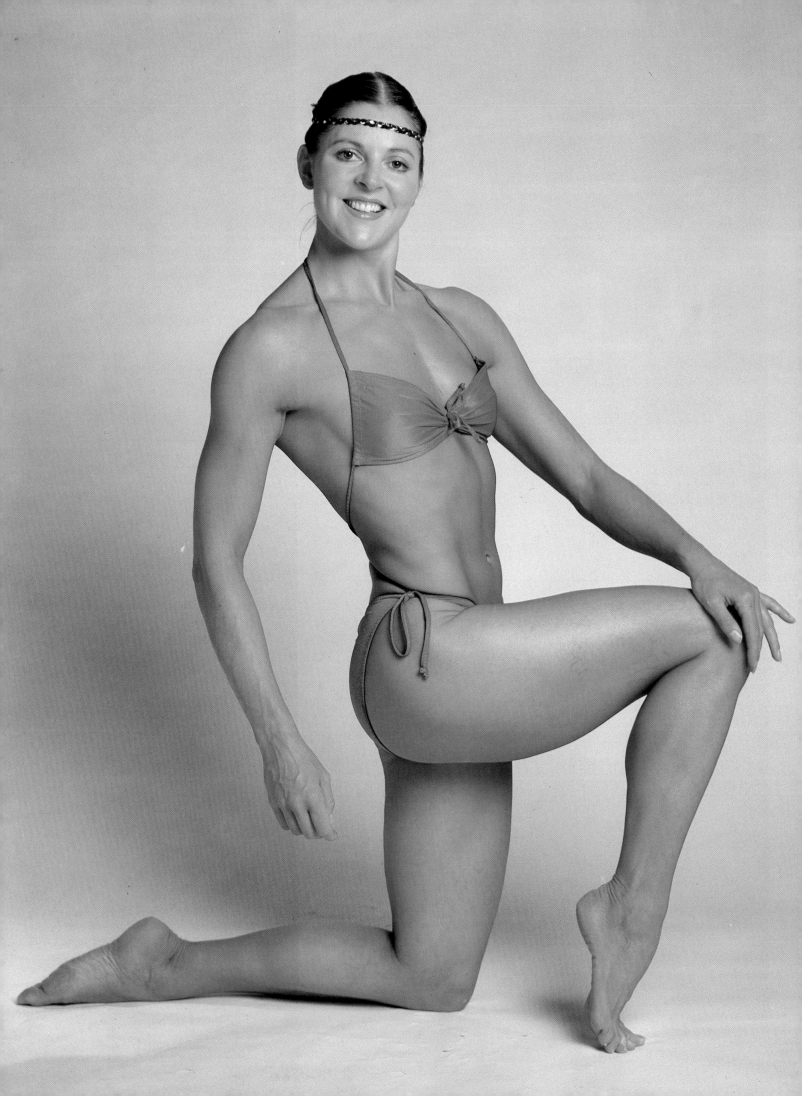

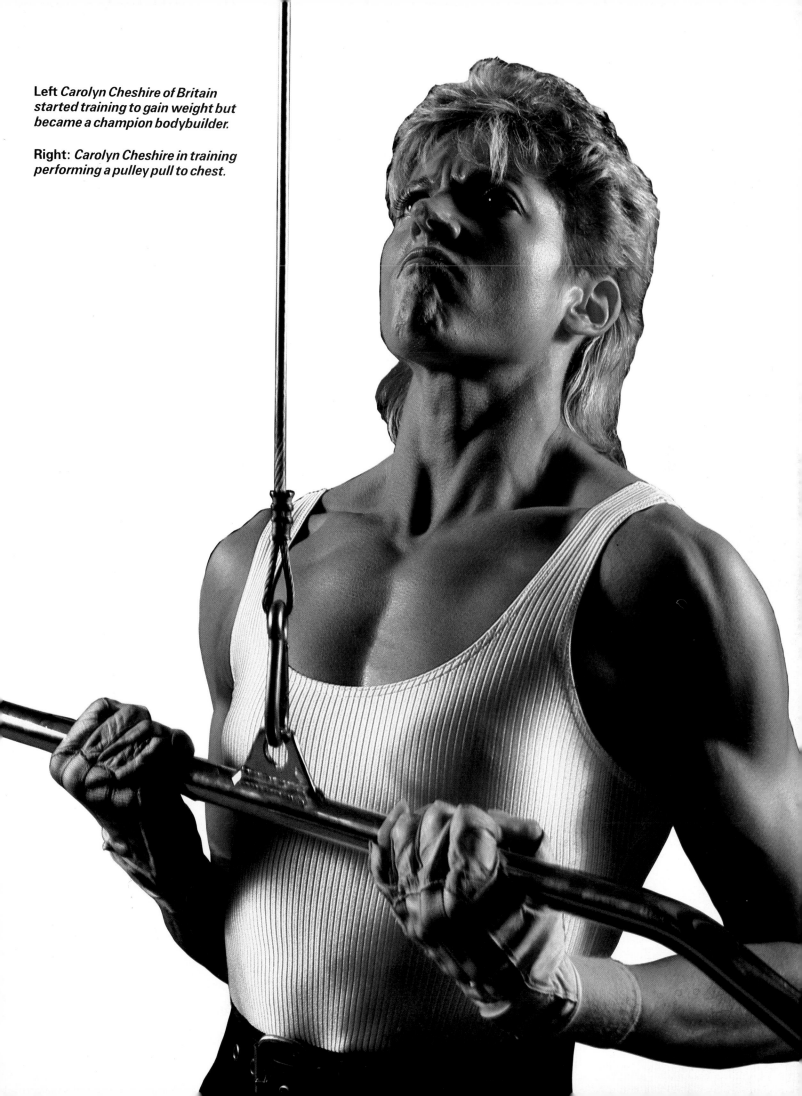

Left *Carolyn Cheshire of Britain started training to gain weight but became a champion bodybuilder.*

Right: *Carolyn Cheshire in training performing a pulley pull to chest.*

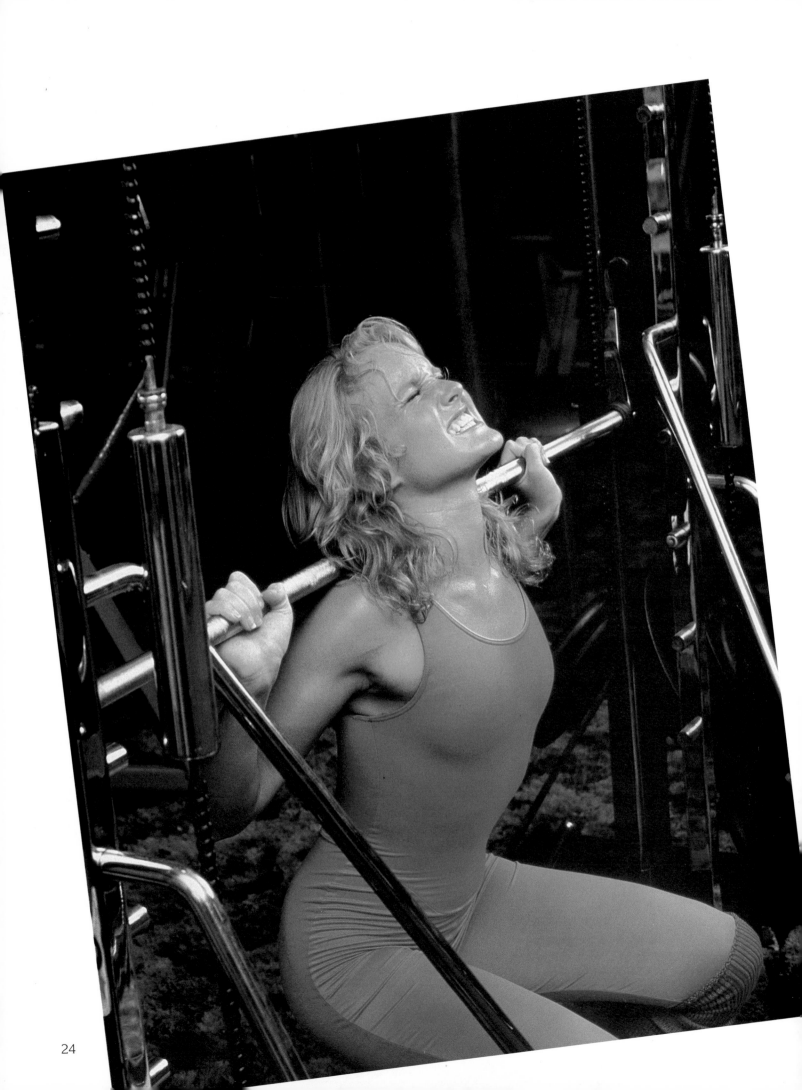

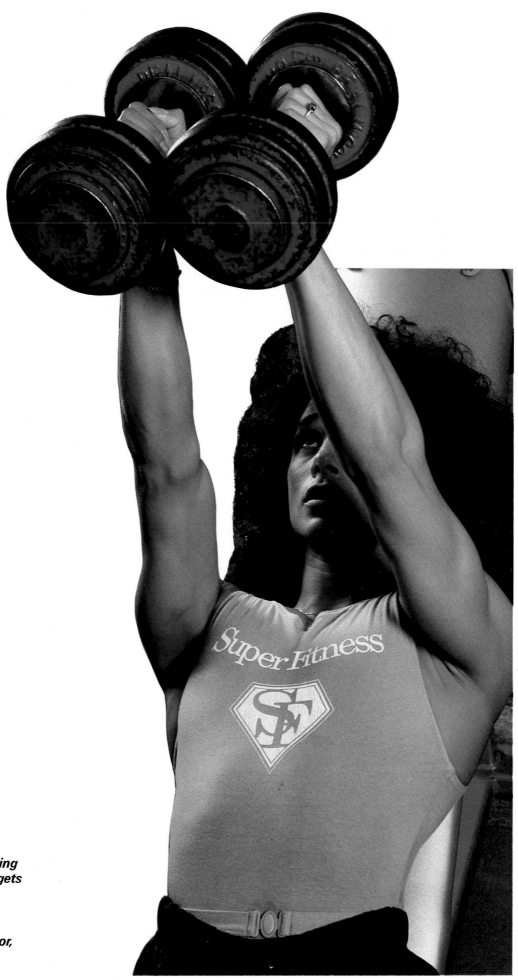

Left *Lorraine Snyder of the USA showing real effort in a bodybuilding workout — the kind of effort that gets results.*

Right *Gladys Portugues, a top American bodybuilding competitor, concentrates on getting those dumbells up high.*

25

SENSIBLE EATING

More books and magazine articles have been written on diet than on almost any other subject. And possibly more nonsense has been written on the subject of diet than on practically any other aspect of human health. It is not surprising that the average woman, bewildered by conflicting advice in every book or magazine she picks up, begins to wonder if the so-called experts really know anything at all. Read them by all means, but then draw your own conclusions when you have tried bodybuilding exercises to go with your diet.

Most of us eat too much. That is a fairly safe statement to make on a subject which bristles with contradictions. The trouble is that we don't eat the right foods. Amazing though it may sound, it is quite possible for a fat person to be suffering from malnutrition.

Many people like to try the latest dietary fad. Some of these diets are cranky but harmless. Others, though, are positively dangerous if followed for any length of time. Many a woman, determined to lose pounds quickly, will willingly reduce herself to near starvation, ruin her health, shred her nerves and, in the process, lose whatever good looks she may have possessed.

Let's use the common sense we were all given at birth. Don't go on any rigid diet unless your doctor recommends it. Sensible eating, combined with regular exercise, is all the average woman needs for health and good looks.

You require different foods to supply the body's varying needs. You must have food to supply fuel for energy and warmth, to build up new tissue and repair old tissue, and to regulate the substances which control the complex machinery of the body.

Certain foods are essential. You need them whether you want to lose or gain weight, or remain the same. Without them you will not be healthy. The essential items of our diet are proteins, carbohydrates, fats, vitamins, minerals and water.

Proteins

The word *protein* means 'first' and is an indication of the importance of the foods within this group. Proteins help to replace and repair the muscular tissue broken down by normal bodily functions. They are the main sources of energy and certain essential minerals.

The best protein foods are milk, eggs, fish, poultry, cheese (especially cottage cheese), and lean meat. To a lesser degree protein is also contained in vegetables, particularly beans, peas, carrots, spinach and cabbage. Soya beans and soya flour are the main constituents of most proprietary protein foods.

With the exception of milk and some cheeses, none of these foods is particularly high in calories. Make sure that your daily diet contains an adequate amount of at least two or three of these items. They are essential to health.

Milk is considered to be the most nearly perfect food. It provides babies with all their nourishment but it is not in itself an adequate diet for an adult. Even so, a pint of milk can provide a quarter of your daily protein requirement. The equivalent would be one good portion of fish or lean meat or two eggs.

Carbohydrates

These supply the body's fuel and are found mainly in sugars and starches.

Most people tend to take too much carbohydrate in the form of bread, cake, pastry and potatoes. But beware of any diet which is completely deficient in carbohydrate; it will make you listless and lifeless. Wholemeal bread is an excellent source.

The sugars in your diet will come from honey, syrup, fruit and glucose. Natural sugars and molasses are better for you than refined products which are little more than 'empty calories'. Glucose is easily taken into the bloodstream.

Vitamins

The term is derived from the word 'life'. There is still a lot to be learned about vitamins and their effect on the human body. We do know that they are essential to health, and we know the foods in which they are found.

Only very small quantities of vitamins are needed and a well-balanced diet including proteins, carbohydrates and fats will also include them. Some people suffer from vitamin deficiency, and vitamin tablets can put this right. But if you lack vitamins it is a sure warning that something is wrong with your daily diet.

Vitamin A is necessary for general health and growth. Lack of it can lead to rough skin and respiratory troubles. The main sources of vitamin A are liver, leafy vegetables, yellow vegetables, cheese, egg yolk, and fruit.

Vitamin B is a complex substance. Lack of vitamin B leads to fatigue, diseases of the nervous system, mental and digestive troubles and constipation. It is found in lean meat, cereals, beans, cheese and some vegetables. Yeast is a good source and is often prescribed by doctors in tablet form.

Vitamin C, generally known as ascorbic acid, is necessary to guard against anemia, depression, rough skin, poor gums and the common cold. The main sources are citrus fruits, tomatoes and many other pulpy fruits.

Vitamin D is sometimes called the 'sunshine vitamin' because it is formed by the action of ultraviolet light on our skins. Lack of it leads to poor teeth and bone structure and makes us less resistant to colds and infection. It is found in eggs, milk, cream and fish oil. Halibut oil and cod liver oil are well known sources.

Vitamin E is commonly known as the 'vitality and fertility vitamin', which adequately describes its qualities. It can be used in cooking with wheat germ oil, or found in whole grain cereals, lettuce, broccoli and brussels sprouts.

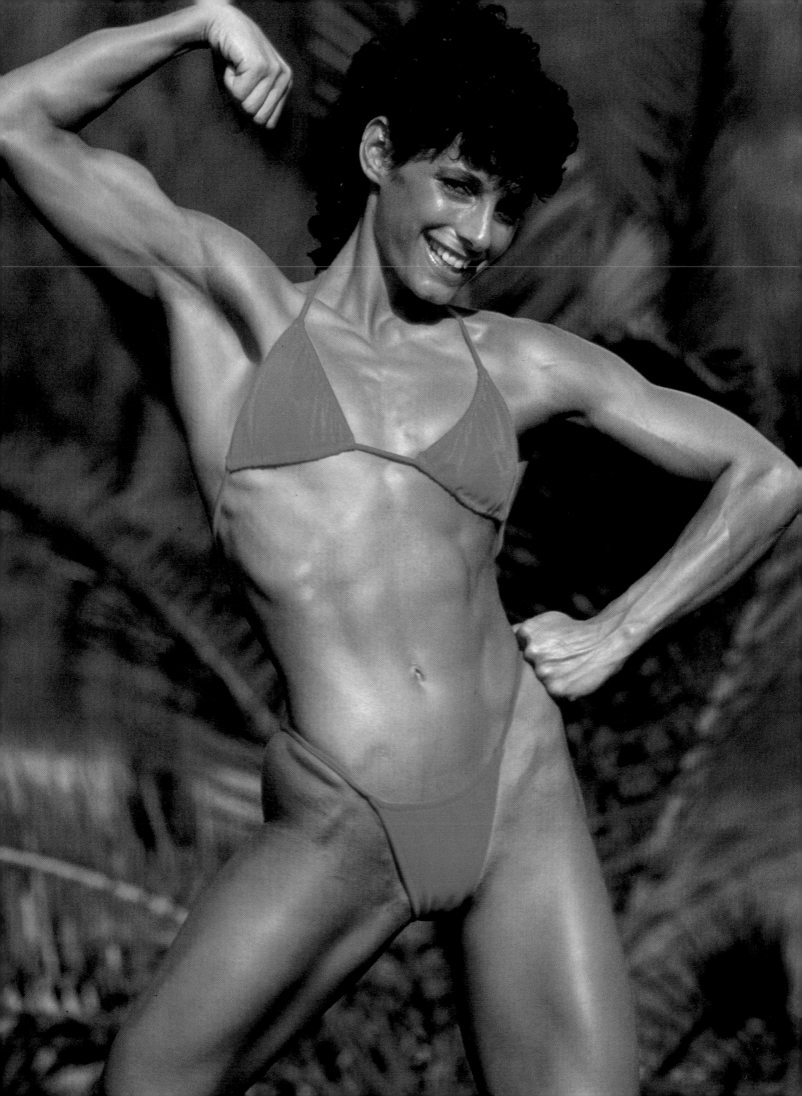

Fats

They are similar in structure to the carbohydrates. Animal sources are butter, meat, bacon and milk. Certain fish — herring and sardine, for instance — are rich in fat. Peanut butter and olive oil are good vegetable sources. There are also small quantities in cheese and eggs.

Minerals

Iron and calcium are essential to the making of blood and bone. They are found in milk, dairy produce, brown bread, vegetables, and fruit. Sulfur and phosphorus are found in many foods, as well as common salt.

There are many other minerals which the body requires to function efficiently, but these are needed in such minute amounts that they should be adequate in a healthy, balanced diet.

Water

About two-thirds of your total bodyweight is fluid. Sufficient water is essential for the proper functioning of the kidneys and to ensure regular elimination.

Do remember that water is not only for washing. It is not very interesting stuff but you should drink at least 3 pints a day. It won't make you fat. And a glass of warm water and lemon first thing every day is better than any branded laxative.

Losing weight

There is no mystery about it at all. Cut down your food intake generally, but make sure that you are getting enough of the essential foods already described in this section to keep you healthy. In other words, follow a good, balanced diet but eat slightly less than you would normally.

Cut down on starches and carbohydrates — less bread, less potatoes, less sugar. Cut down on fats — poached eggs for breakfast instead of fried, cottage cheese instead of cheddar. Eat more fresh food, especially fruit and vegetables.

There is no need to be a martyr. In fact, a diet which makes you feel listless and constantly hungry is guaranteed to fail, since you will be always thinking about food and are much more likely to sneak the odd cookie or abandon the diet altogether. Regulate your diet on these simple lines, perform a bodybuilding routine regularly, and you will reduce gradually and safely.

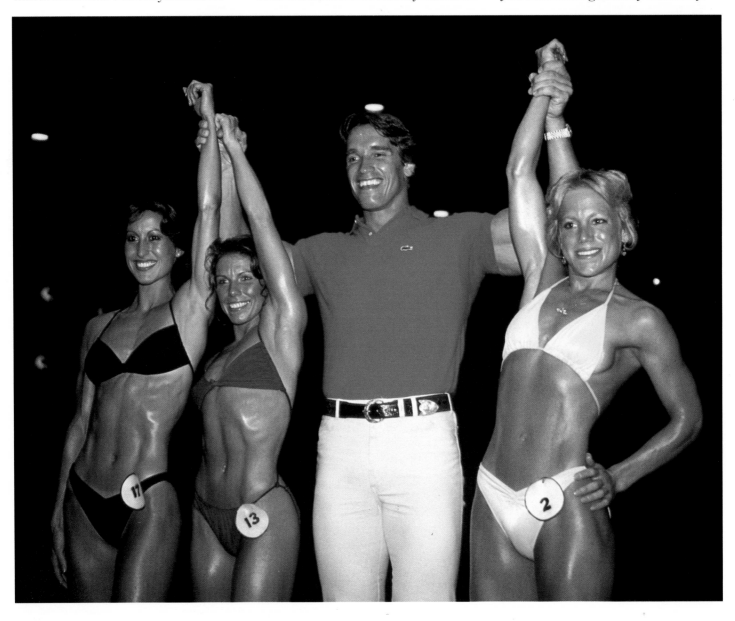

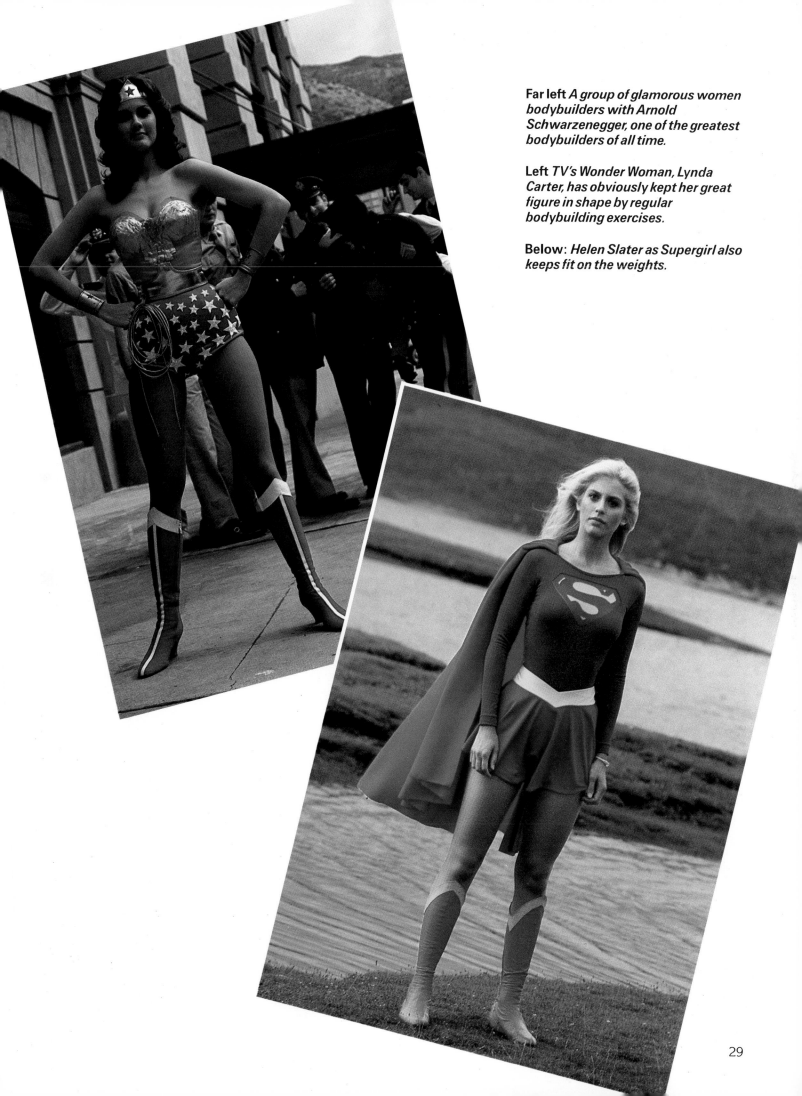

Far left *A group of glamorous women bodybuilders with Arnold Schwarzenegger, one of the greatest bodybuilders of all time.*

Left *TV's Wonder Woman, Lynda Carter, has obviously kept her great figure in shape by regular bodybuilding exercises.*

Below: *Helen Slater as Supergirl also keeps fit on the weights.*

29

Gaining weight

Eat almost anything, but still limit fried foods, pastries, rich cakes, etc.

Include extra milk — at least one pint a day — chocolate, icecream, bananas, extra cheese and eggs, plenty of butter, honey, molasses, nuts, raisins. Olive oil, halibut oil, or cod liver oil and malt can also be taken.

Health foods

So-called health foods are a multi-million dollar business, and every week some new miracle pill appears. Nearly every reputable drugstore has a health food counter, and specialist shops flourish. They sell two main kinds of products: healthy foods, such as wholemeal bread and flours, natural yoghurt, nuts, fruits, and so on; and food supplements, such as vitamin pills, which are designed to supplement your normal diet with essential vitamins and minerals which you may be lacking.

Everyone should eat more healthy foods, rather than the fatty, over-sweet junk foods which comprise such a large proportion of our diet, but most of these are readily available in supermarkets and ordinary shops and probably cost less there. Among the healthiest foods are fresh fruit and vegetables, which really makes the term health food a misnomer.

The majority of normal, healthy people who follow a good balanced diet should obtain all the necessary nutrients from their food without the need for supplements, although they do have an important place in any health plan, and are invaluable for sportspeople and those involved in heavy physical work, and are ideal as an extra tonic to be used after illness, for example.

But what do you take? The variety of food supplements is inexhaustible, as are the makers, and the advertised advantages of some products are unproven. It is therefore wise to use only supplements of proven value. A good protein drink, for example, made with milk, is ideal if you are run down, but remember that too much milk is fattening, so cut the milk if you are trying to lose weight. Wheatgerm capsules are ideal for extra vitamin E, and so on.

Generally speaking, doctors are reticent about the advantages and disadvantages of advertised health foods, probably because there are so many, and they feel that some are phoney. Yet everyone realizes the importance of obtaining essential vitamins — doctors often prescribe extra vitamin B, for example, during convalescence. The important thing is to be sceptical of the so-called 'miracle-workers', but be aware of the advantages and the place of recognized food supplements in your diet.

In general, most common food supplements are harmless, but you should always follow recommended doses. Most people will not feel the need to use them, but for athletes, in special circumstances, and when fresh vegetables and good foods are expensive or hard to obtain, dietary supplements can play an important role in keeping you healthy.

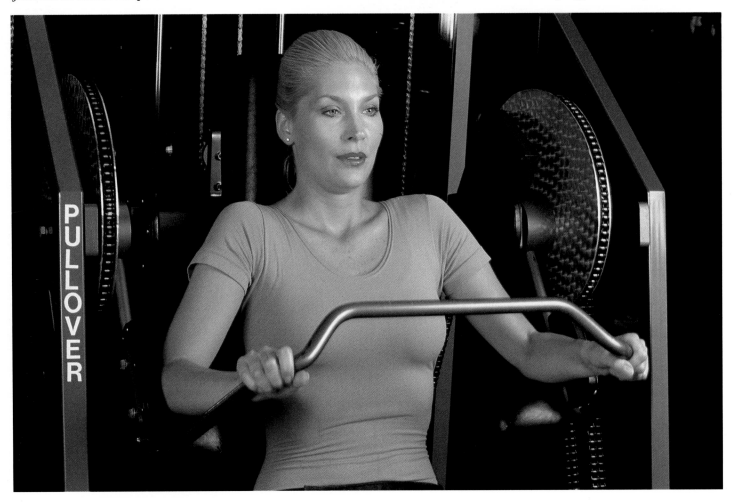

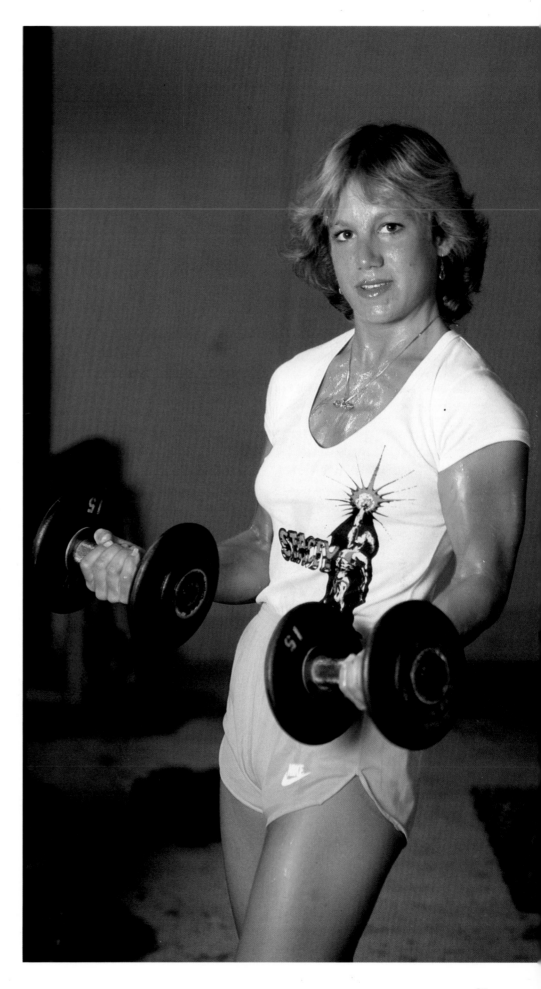

Left *Marjorie Harris training on the widely-used Nautilus equipment.*

Right *Paula Harris performing a two-hands dumbell curl. This upper arm exercise is for more advanced bodybuilders.*

The secrets of good eating

Nobody can tell you exactly what to eat and when to eat it; individuals vary considerably. One woman may thrive on two large meals a day. Another woman may need frequent small snacks. But it is a good idea to try to eat at the same times every day. This can be difficult, but the stomach is very much a creature of habit. If you possibly can, indulge your stomach on this point.

Avoid nibbling between meals. Skipping a wholesome breakfast and then having two cookies with your coffee is no good for anyone. Also try to avoid heavy meals late in the evening, because your body does not have time to use up the calories.

Take some care in the preparation of food. Don't overcook it and destroy its natural goodness. Avoid frying — grill, steam, poach or bake instead. Don't eat warmed-up leftovers — fresh, well-cooked food has far more nutritional value.

Give yourself time to eat a meal. Food should be eaten slowly and well chewed. Rushed meals are one of the greatest single causes of digestive troubles and constipation.

There is no such thing as a miracle-working diet that will solve your health and weight problems in a couple of weeks. If you have been following a bad diet for years, you cannot expect your body to adjust overnight, so the sooner you start the better — and don't give up. If your diet is unbalanced, too high in fats, refined carbohydrates and junk foods, then the only answer is to change it.

Eat according to the suggestions made in this section, watch those fats and carbohydrates, perform the bodybuilding exercises regularly, and health and figure beauty will be yours.

It will take a little time before you begin to see results, but they will certainly come. And as the months go by, and you check your progress in the mirror and on the bathroom scales — as well as simply by the way you feel — you will come to agree that sensible eating and a little scientific exercise are not such bad things after all.

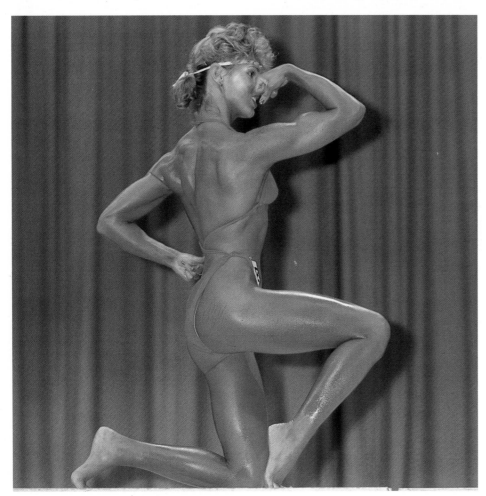

Left *This pose is popular with many international bodybuilding contestants.*

Right *Corina Everson of the USA displays fine upper body muscularity.*

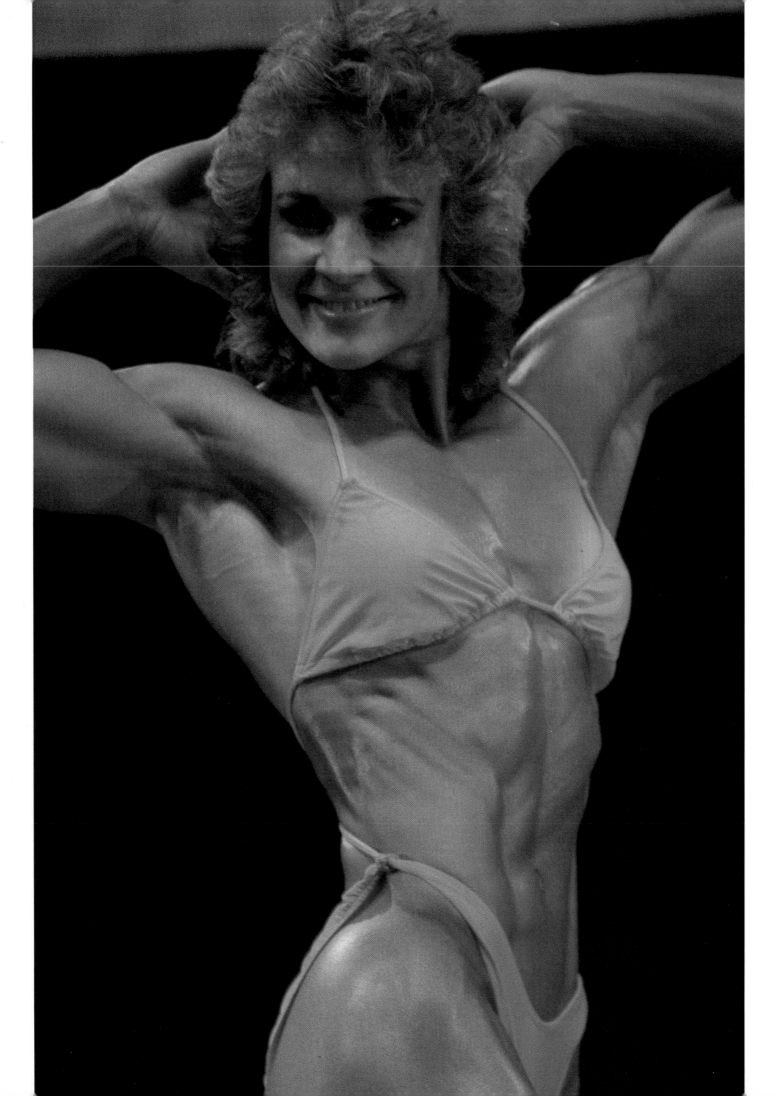

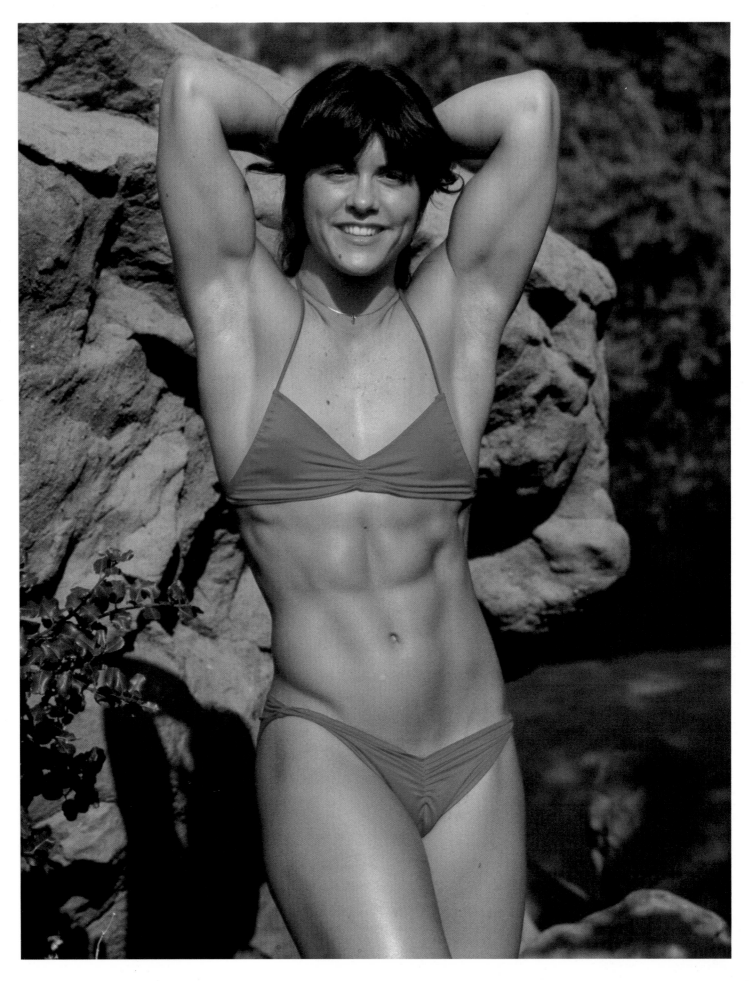

34

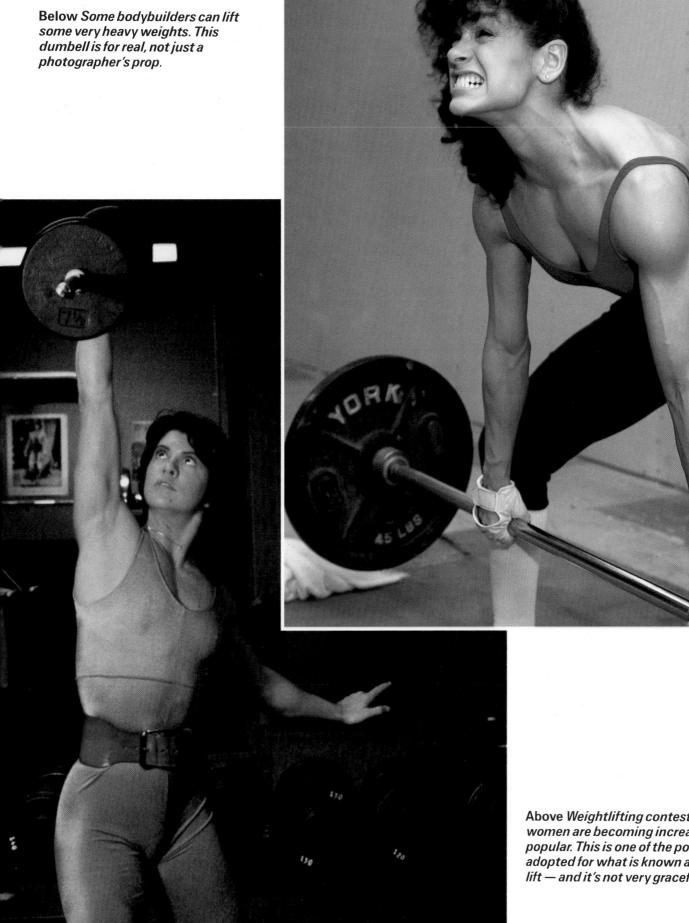

Left *Penny Price of the USA looks healthy and happy — all thanks to positive bodybuilding.*

Below *Some bodybuilders can lift some very heavy weights. This dumbell is for real, not just a photographer's prop.*

Above *Weightlifting contests for women are becoming increasingly popular. This is one of the positions adopted for what is known as a dead lift — and it's not very graceful!*

35

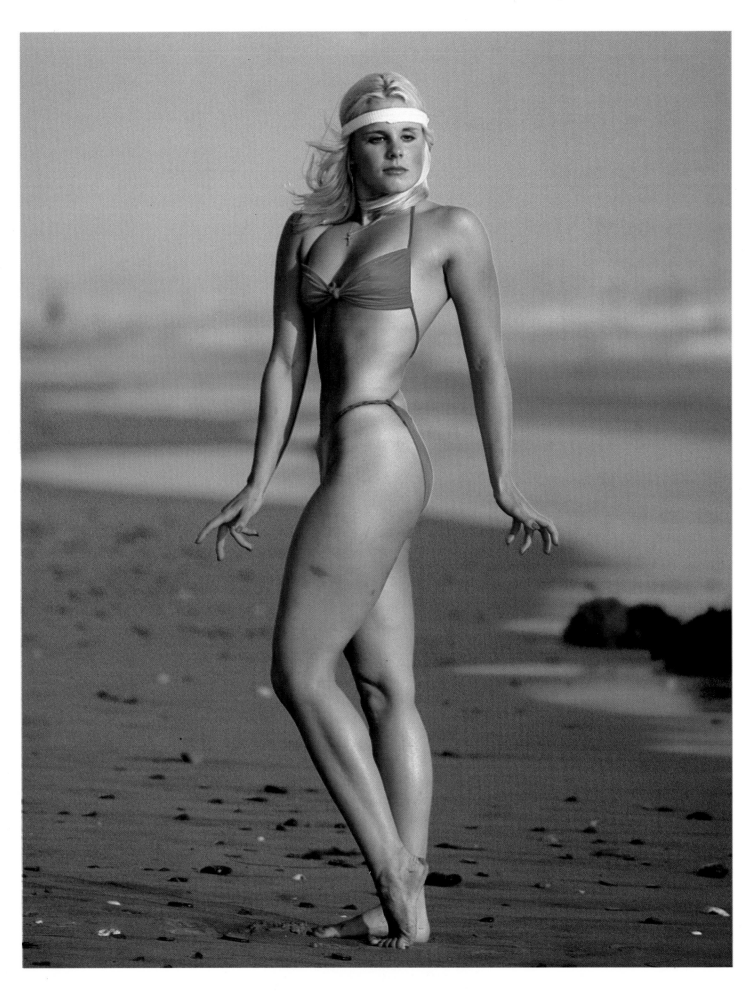

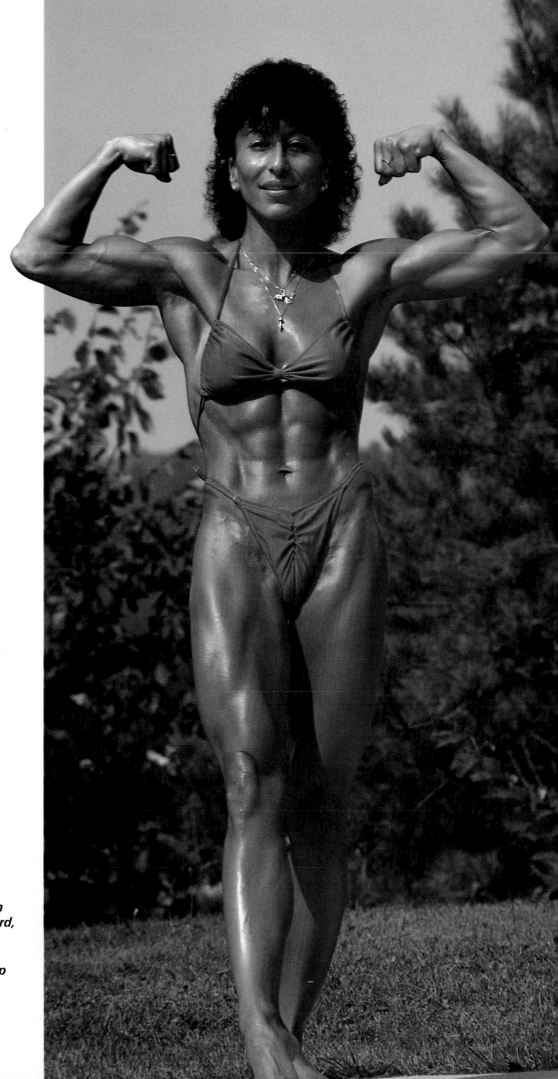

Left *The perfect figure of today can also be yours. Remember: train hard, look great.*

Right *A double biceps pose by a top physique girl. Muscularity can be yours — if you want it.*

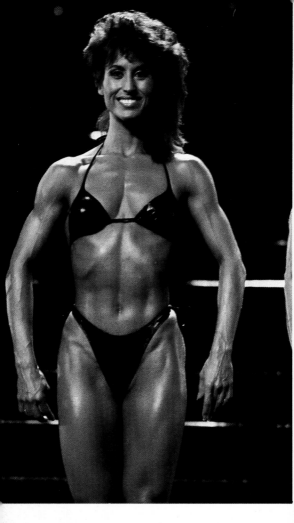

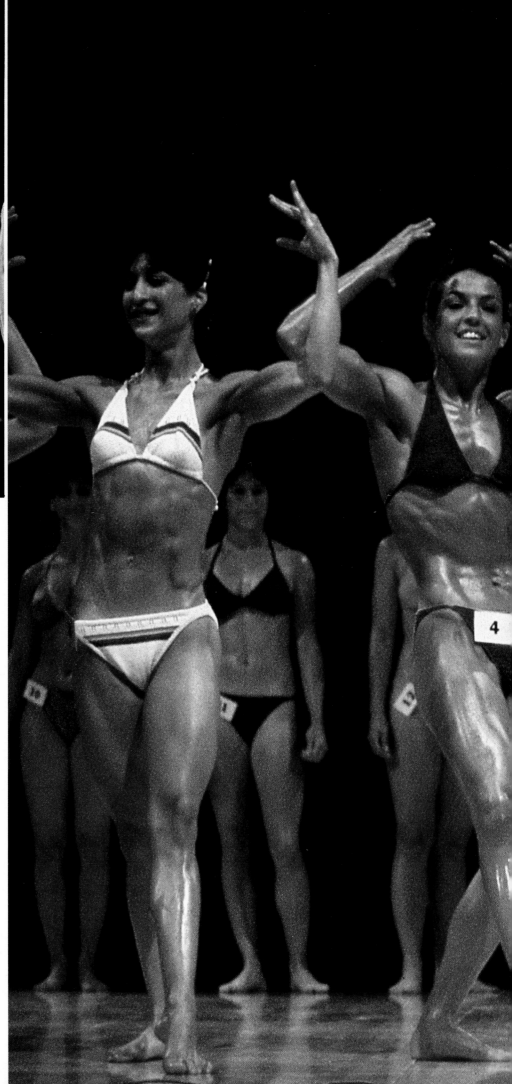

Above *Bodybuilder Rachel McLish of the USA.*

Right *Competitors display before the judges in a bodybuilding contest.*

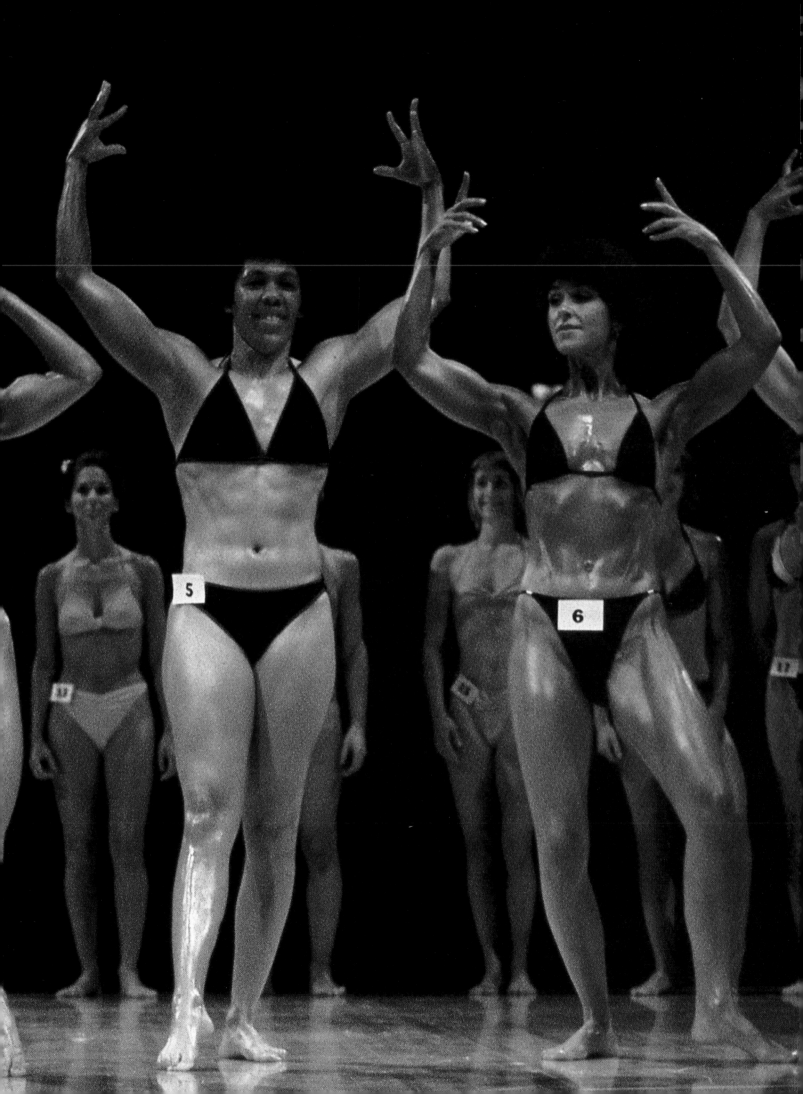

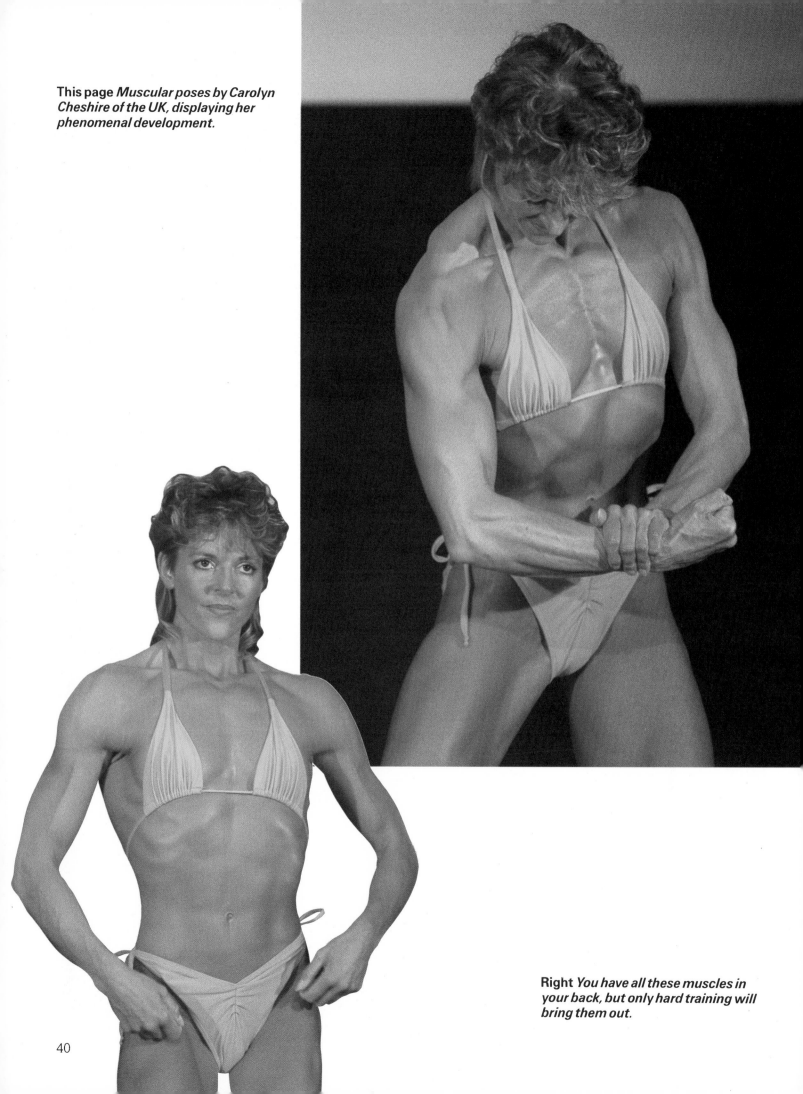

This page *Muscular poses by Carolyn Cheshire of the UK, displaying her phenomenal development.*

Right *You have all these muscles in your back, but only hard training will bring them out.*

40

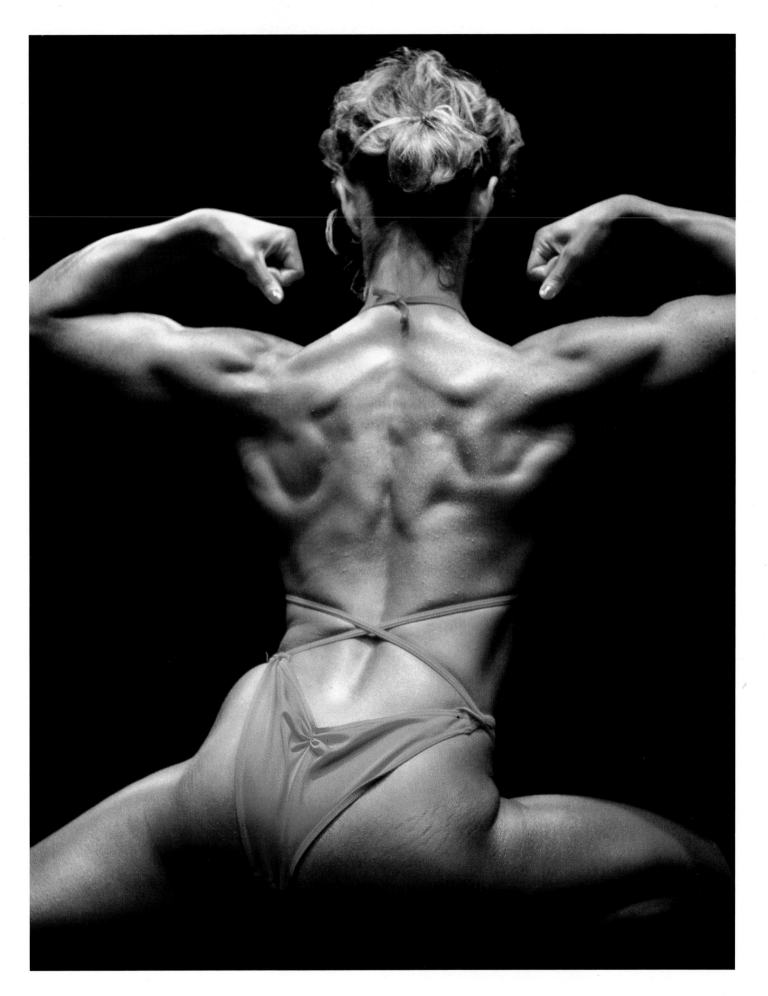

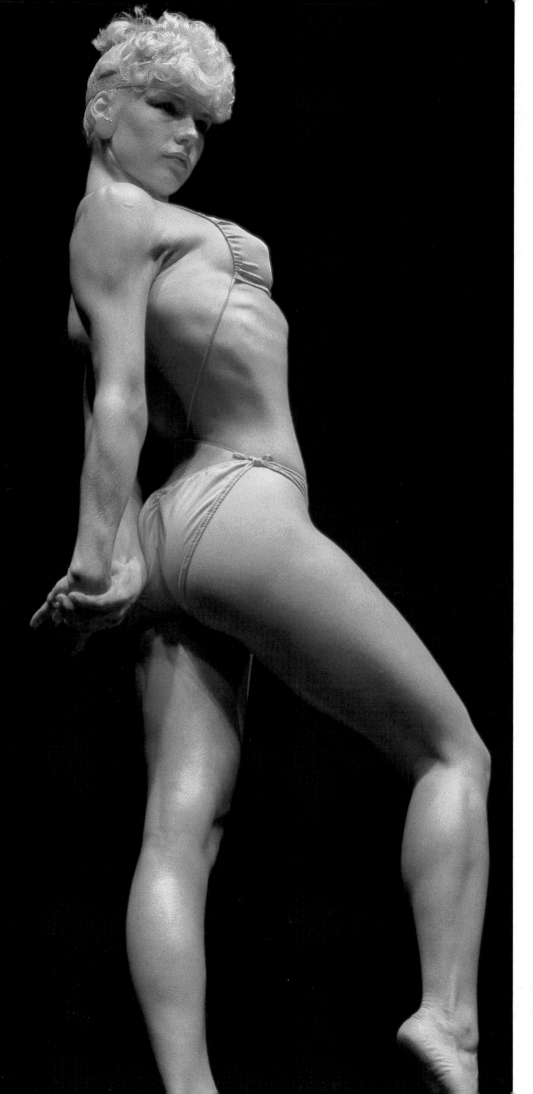

Left *A typical pose from a women's bodybuilding contest.*

Right *Mary Scott of Scotland can boast two fine achievements. She is a top bodybuilder and also the mother of three children.*

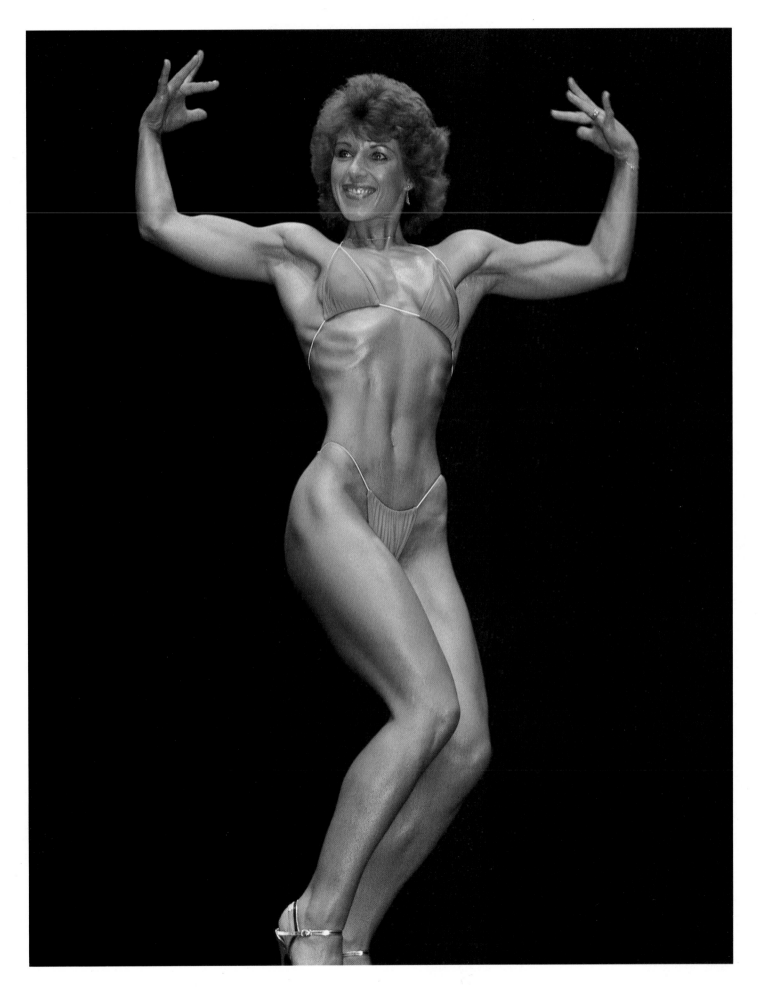

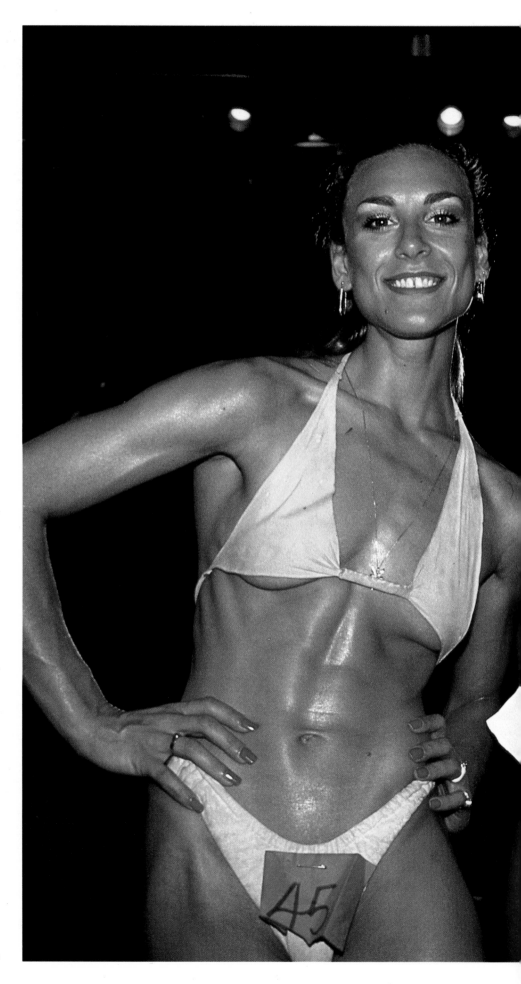

A trio of glamorous muscle girls in an American women's physique contest.

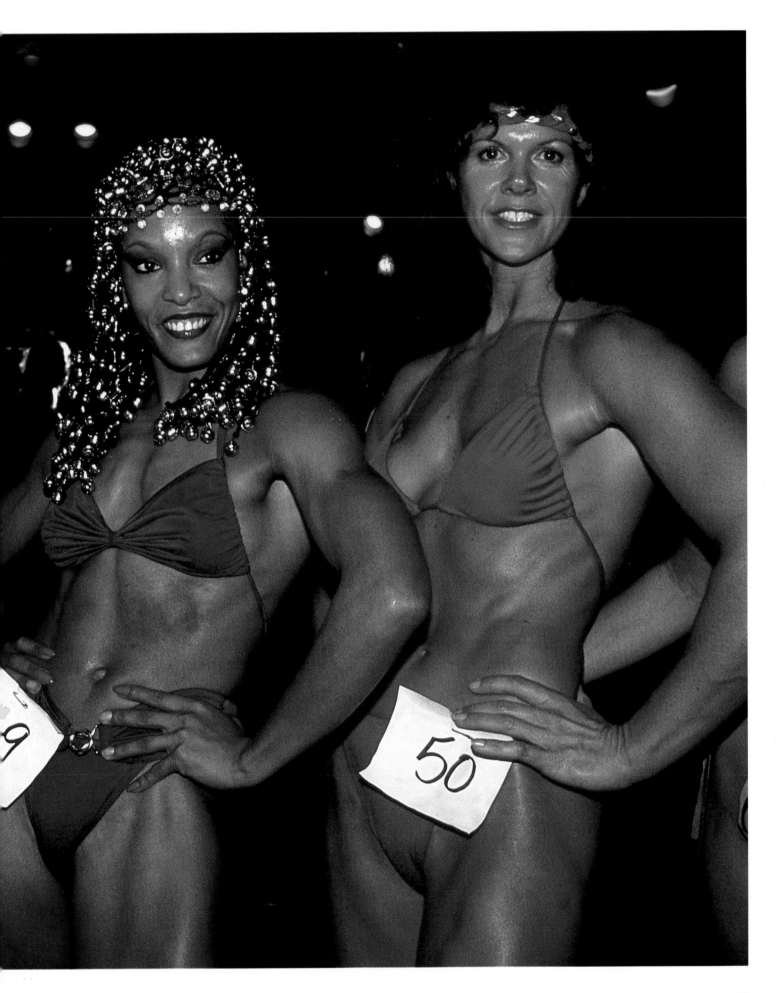

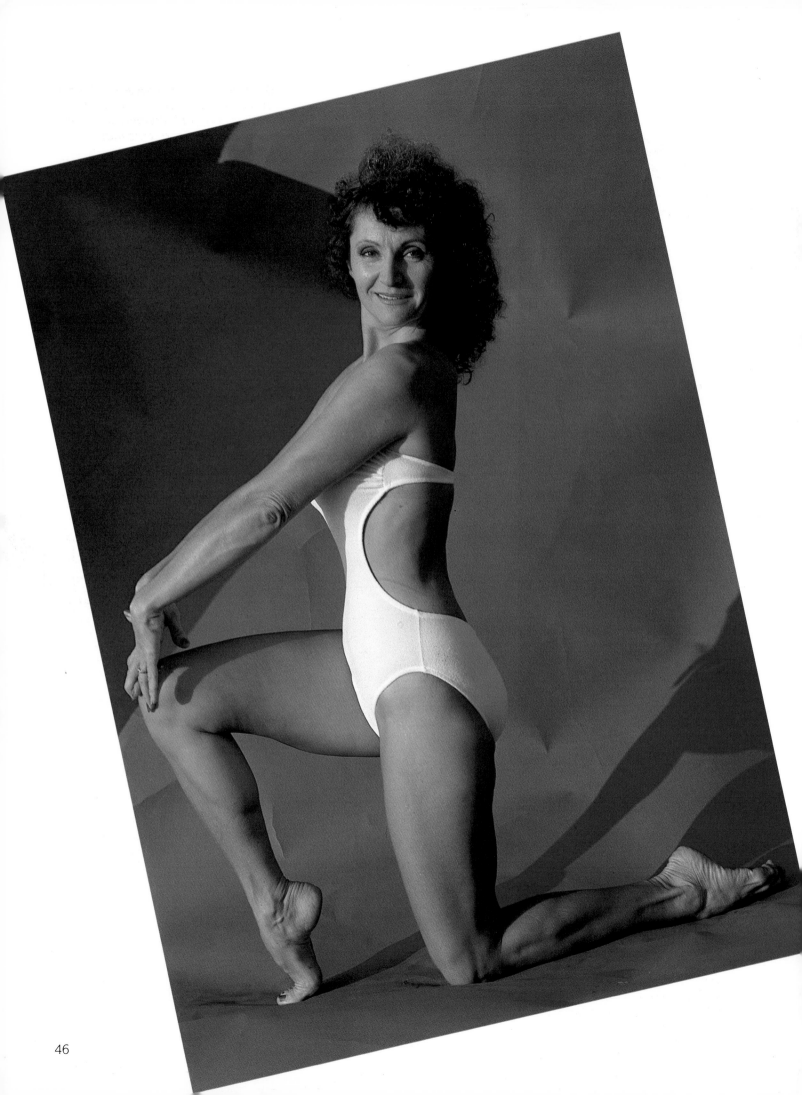

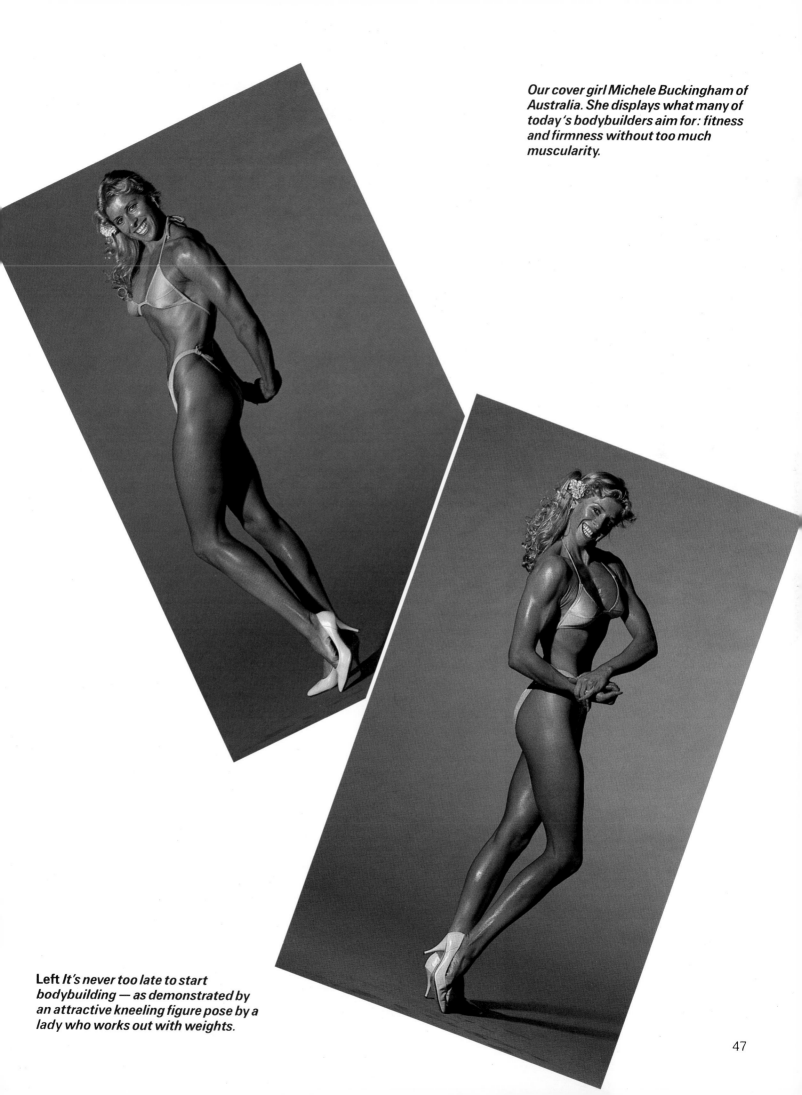

Our cover girl Michele Buckingham of Australia. She displays what many of today's bodybuilders aim for: fitness and firmness without too much muscularity.

Left *It's never too late to start bodybuilding — as demonstrated by an attractive kneeling figure pose by a lady who works out with weights.*

47

FREESTANDING EXERCISES FOR TONING-UP

Any type of regular exercise can do nothing but good for you. Any sport is enjoyable mentally, physically and socially. But for many people sport is an impossibility because of lack of facilities, the time involved, cost, etc. However, the great present-day boom in health clubs and gymnasiums, with their accessibility and comparatively low cost, leaves you with no excuse not to do something about it yourself.

Better still, bodybuilding can be done at home, either alone or with a training partner. It can be shared with a friend, male or female. It is comparatively cheap, it is progressive, and the equipment does not wear out and can be added to as you progress. Above all, it does not take up much time.

Whether you train at home or at a health studio, the ideal is to train three times a week, for about an hour, or at least twice a week, with two or three days separating the workouts. A health club is ideal, provided you get good instruction. On the other hand, after a few months, you should be quite capable of making up your own work schedules.

There are very few sports you can carry on alone, but bodybuilding is one of them. A training companion can be valuable, but only if they will stick it like you intend to do.

Modern health clubs may seem expensive, but they are not if you use them regularly and take full advantage of what they have to offer. Where else could you pass the time away for as little and do yourself a lot of good at the same time? You will also be meeting other people of both sexes with similar interests.

What to wear

There are so many attractive new types of leotards, without legs and with full-length leg coverings, that you are spoilt for choice. There are also the many new types of tracksuits, also ideal for training. Whatever you choose, it must be made of flexible material so that it in no way restricts your movements. And there must be no constrictions round the waist.

If you are heavy-busted, you must have the right support, as long as it is not tight and restrictive, with too many straps.

Even in summer you must start off warm. It is no use coming into a gym that may be draughty until you have loosened and warmed up. Light socks, preferably not nylon, are best, with a very light ballet or gymnastic-type slip-on shoe. This is far better than the fashionable heavy and rather hard type of sports shoe worn for jogging and so many other sports.

In winter, leg warmers of various kinds are very useful. Don't let yourself grow cold during your workout — this too often results from hanging about between exercises.

Bare feet may be ideal at home in summer, but not in a health club. Most clubs will not allow bare feet because of the risk of picking up or spreading germs through dust on floors, however clean they may be kept.

Freestanding exercises

The following exercises can keep you fit and well, even without the added benefits of exercises with weights. All the freestanding exercises are illustrated in Section II.

Gym bicycle

This is a great way to start any workout program. It will get the heart and circulation working correctly before the more strenuous bodybuilding exercises begin. Spend two or three minutes on the cycle, adjusting the resistance as you become fitter.

Arms raise forward and upward

Stand astride with your arms at your sides, fingers pointed, thumbs to the front. Swing your arms forward and upward, smoothly and without any body movement. Try and get your arms straight above your head in line with your ears. This may be difficult at first if you are stiff in the shoulders or have bad posture. It is very important to breathe in through your mouth as you swing your arms gently upwards, and out as you lower them. Repeat 10 times.

Arms circling

As a progression of the above complete the circle of the arms by taking them backwards, and back to a starting position. Try and brush your ears with the inside of your upper arm. This is a very good posture exercise, and a bust improver. Repeat 10 times.

Sidebends in neck rest position

Cup your hands behind your neck, keeping your shoulders well back and not allowing them to come forward in any way. Quite briskly bend from side to side as far as you can, as long as there is no forward lean of the body. Let your head and neck move freely, do not hold them stiff. Breathe normally and make the movement continuous to left and right. Repeat to count of 20.

Trunk forward bend to reach alternative instep

Stand feet astride, hands at your sides. Reach down to touch the opposite instep with both hands. Go through the upright position each time and swing over to the opposite side. Try 10 repetitions in a complete circular movement on each side. Breathe normally. As a progression when you are supple enough and can grasp your ankle with both hands, pull your head towards the angle two or three times on each move.

Cat stretch

Support your weight on your arms in the front support position, legs

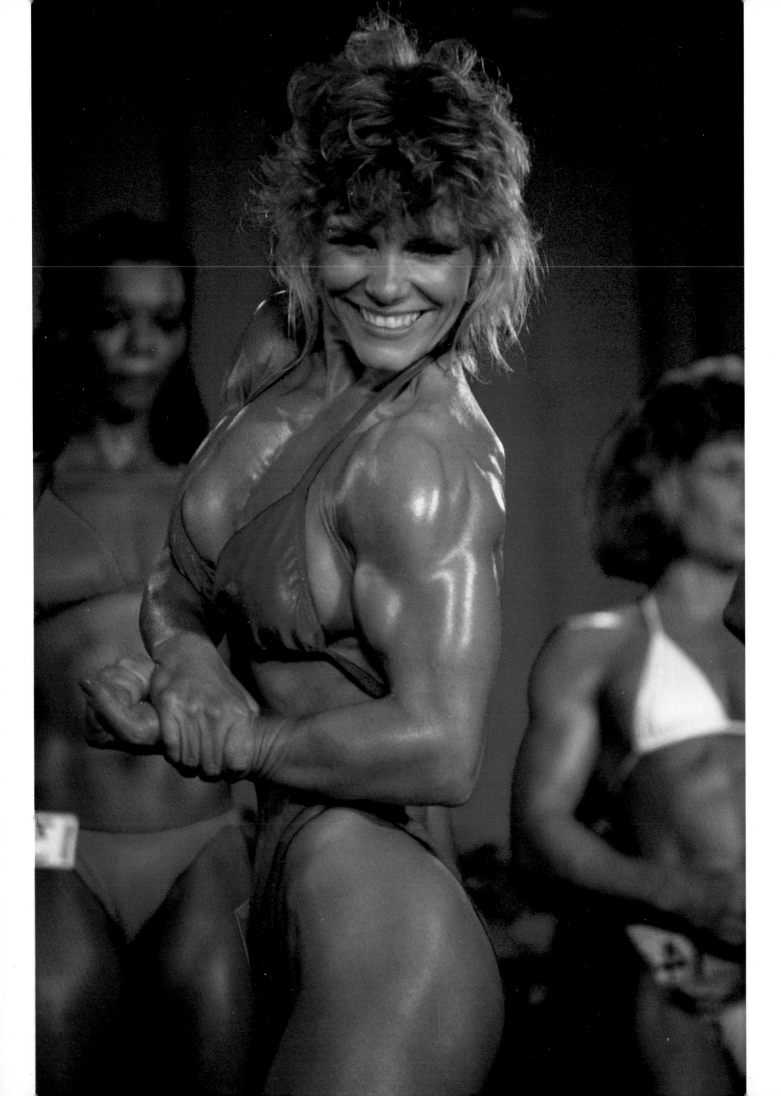

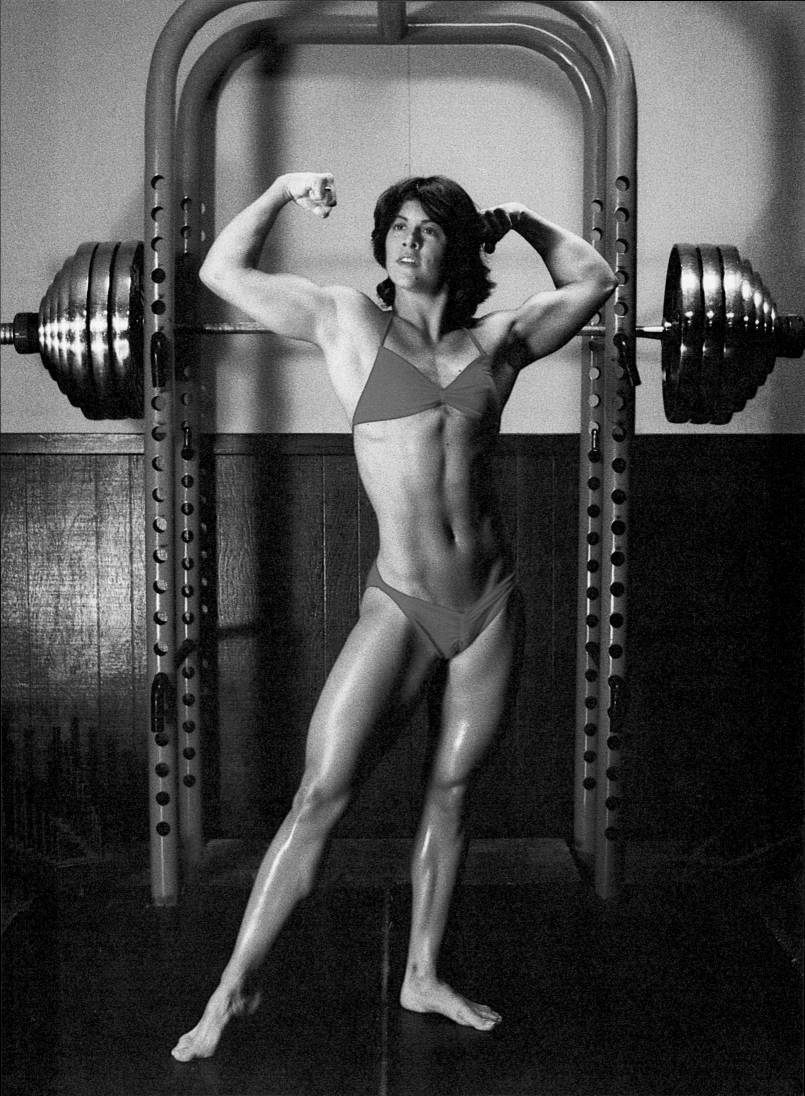

straight, body in a straight line from head to toe, no sag in the middle. Without bending your arms, lower your hips and legs to touch the floor, lifting your head as high as possible. Breathe in as you lower your hips, out as you return to the starting position. Repeat 10 times.

As a progression, you can also raise your hips as high as possible, making an inverted V position, trying to put your heels on the floor. You see cats stretching in this way.

Lying alternate knee raise to chest

Lie on your back, hands at sides, legs straight, and toes pointed. Raise alternate knees high to your chest, but do not move your head. Keep the other leg straight. After some practice this can be done fairly rapidly. Breathe normally. When fit and your waist has returned to normal, progress by raising both knees to your chest. Later in the neck rest position, you can progress to legs raising, and so on.

Sitting trunk forward bend to reach toes

Sit with legs straight, swing your arms towards your toes, trying to reach them without bending your legs. Breathe in before you reach forward, out as you return to the sitting position. Later, reach forward in beats of three. A progression is the sit-ups from the prone position, but you will need something to anchor your feet, or a partner to hold them down.

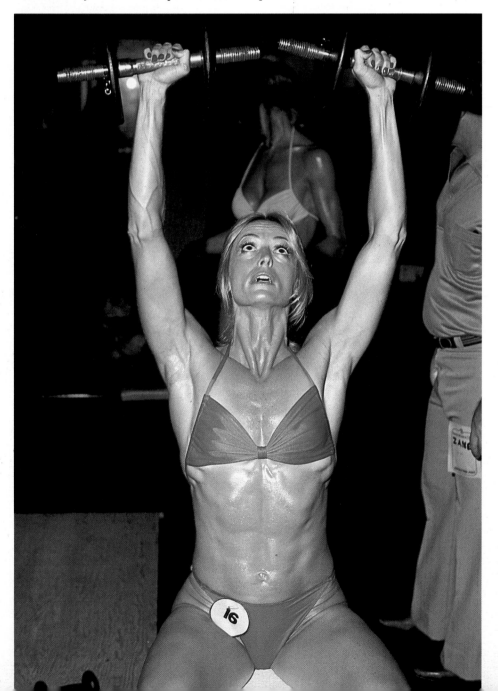

Previous page *This stunning 'side chest pose' shows the results of hard training.*

Far left *A classical 'double biceps' pose.*

Left *Dumbell exercises are a basic ingredient of all bodybuilding programs.*

Hyperextensions

Lie flat on the floor with your arms in the neck rest position, i.e., clasped behind your head. Forcing your arms back, raise your head and shoulders off the floor as high as possible. Breathe in as you lift, out as you lower. Repeat 10 times.

A progression is to try and grasp your ankles with both hands and pull strongly, making your body into a curve. Breathe in as you pull, out as you relax.

This is a wonderful exercise for strengthening the back and getting rid of backaches, as long as you do not have a specific back injury.

Squats (knees bend)

Stand feet astride about 12 ins apart. You may need a block about three inches high under your heels for this. But if you are supple enough to do the exercise without a block, do so. It will compensate for wearing high heels. Quick knees bend and stretch until your thighs are parallel with the floor. Keep your back flat, and do not sag in any way. Breathe in just before the knees bend, out as you come to the upright position.
Repeat 10 times.

Side kicks

Lie sideways on the floor, supporting your chin in one hand and with your elbow on the floor and your free leg straight. Kick the free leg sideways vigorously. This is very good for the inside of the thighs. Try 10 on each side. This exercise can also be performed standing.

Relaxation

Every training program, whether freestanding or with weights, should finish with a minute or two in the relaxed position to restore the systems — breathing, heart, etc — to normal. Lie on your back, arms at your sides, palms of your hands on the floor. Raise your knees well up, keeping the soles of your feet on the floor. Try and take all the hollows out of your back and touch the whole of your spine on the floor by imagining that you are tucking your bottom in.

Close your eyes and breathe deeply through your nose, filling your lungs to capacity. Breathe out slowly, until you feel you can breathe out no more air, but just try to do so. Lie for about three minutes and relax completely. This is a very valuable finale to your workout.

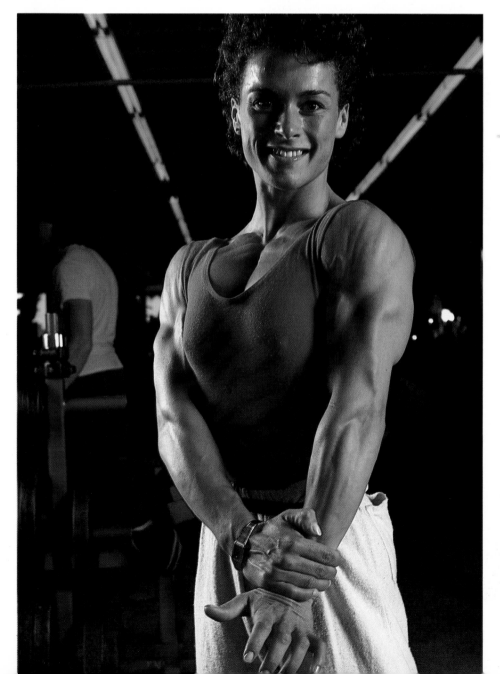

Left *Top European bodybuilder Erika Mes of Holland, a pioneer of women's physique contests and winner of many titles.*

Right *Karen Stevenson of the UK demonstrates that bodybuilding for women is not all about bulging muscles.*

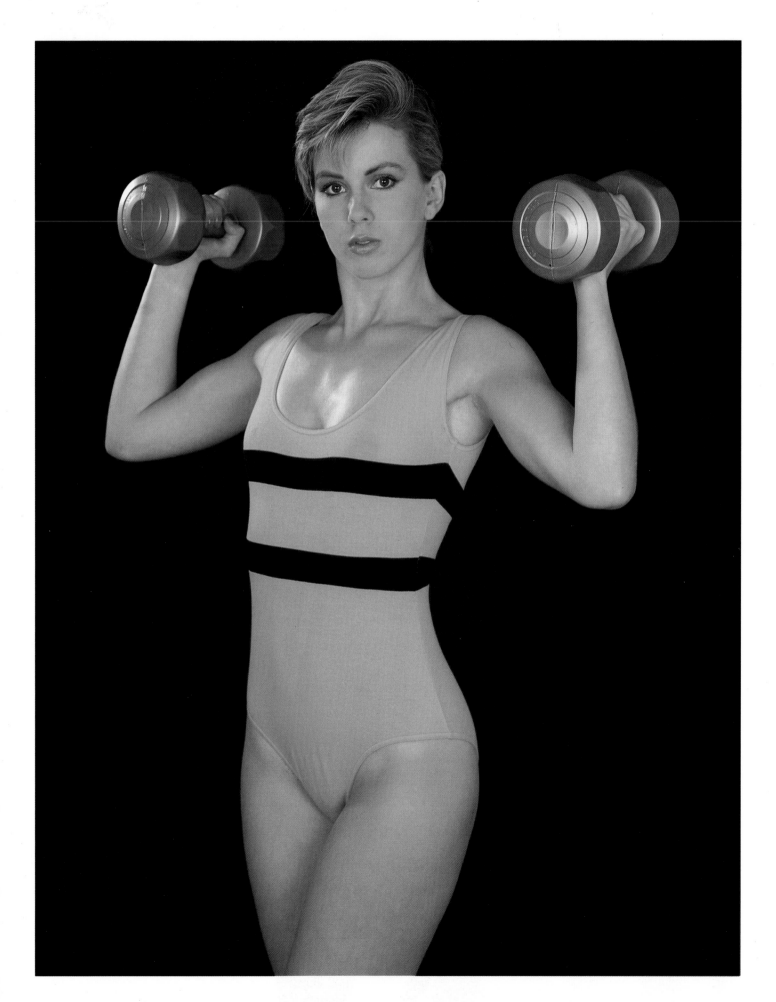

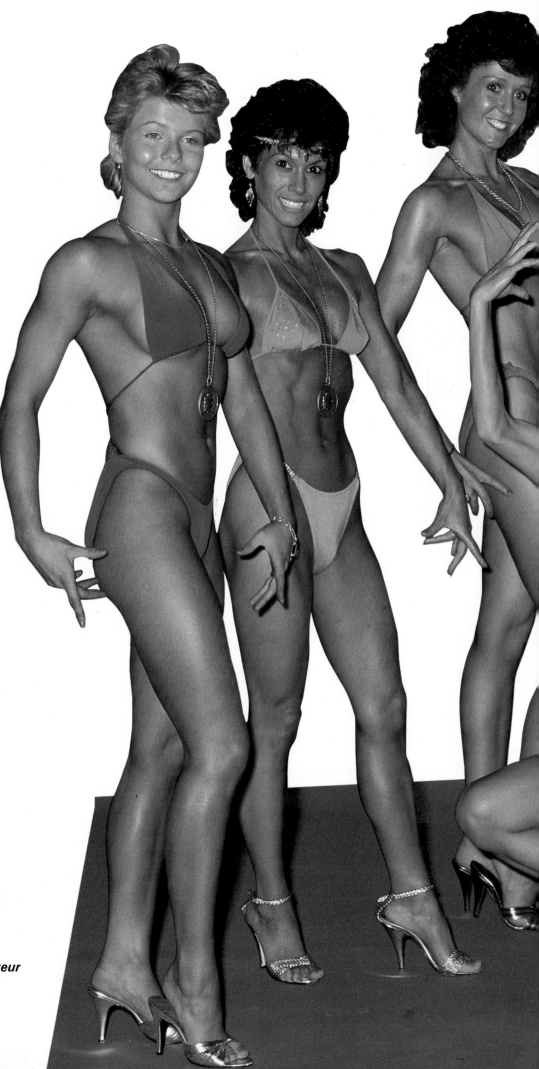

A group of NABBA (National Amateur Bodybuilders' Association) Miss Britain finalists.

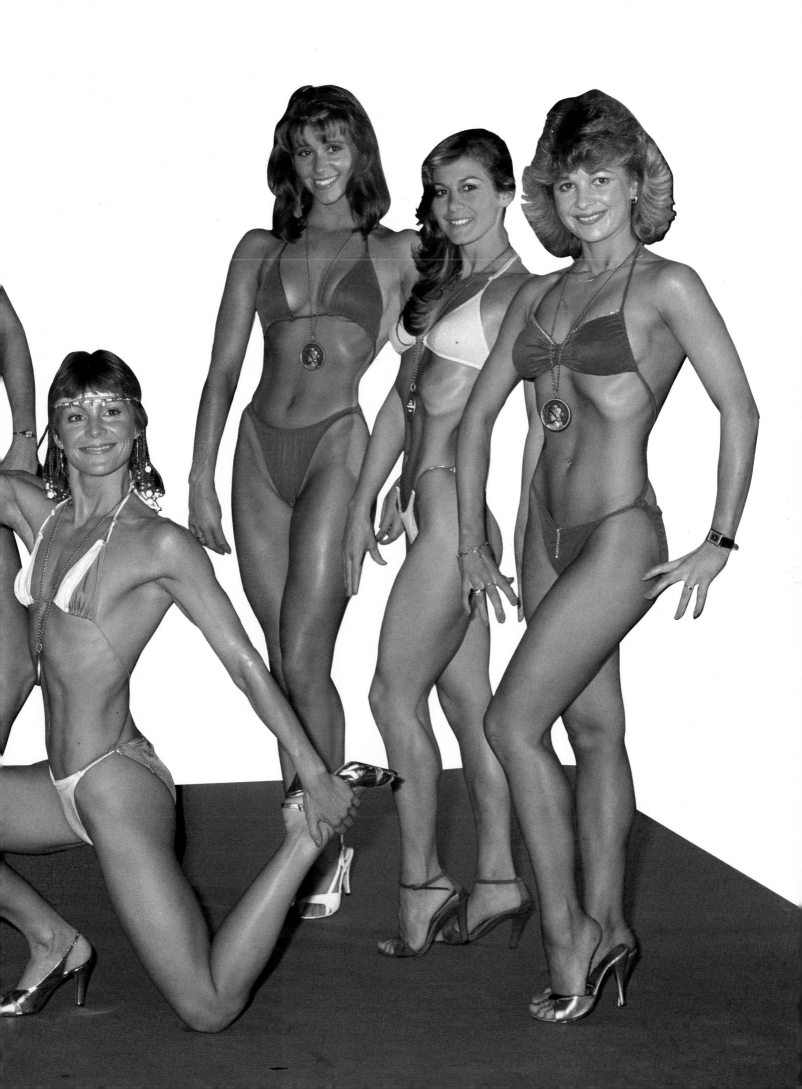

This page *These graceful poses demand balance, control — and a lot of practice.*

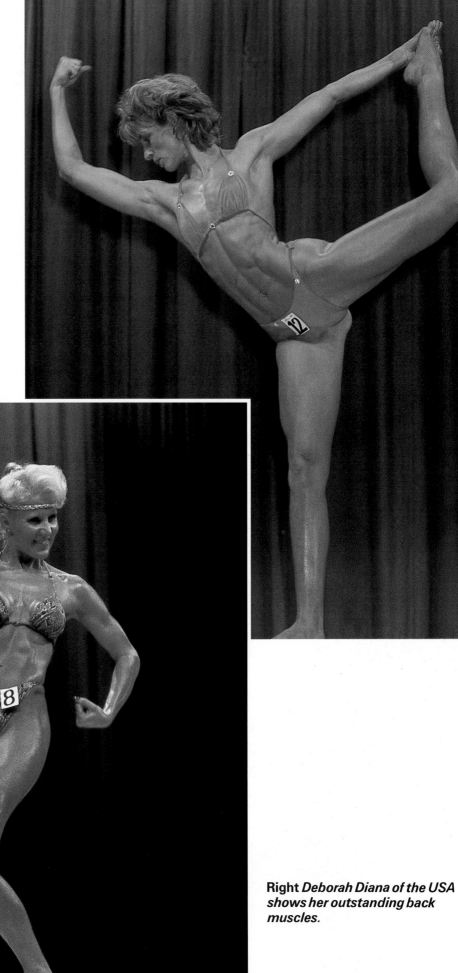

Right *Deborah Diana of the USA shows her outstanding back muscles.*

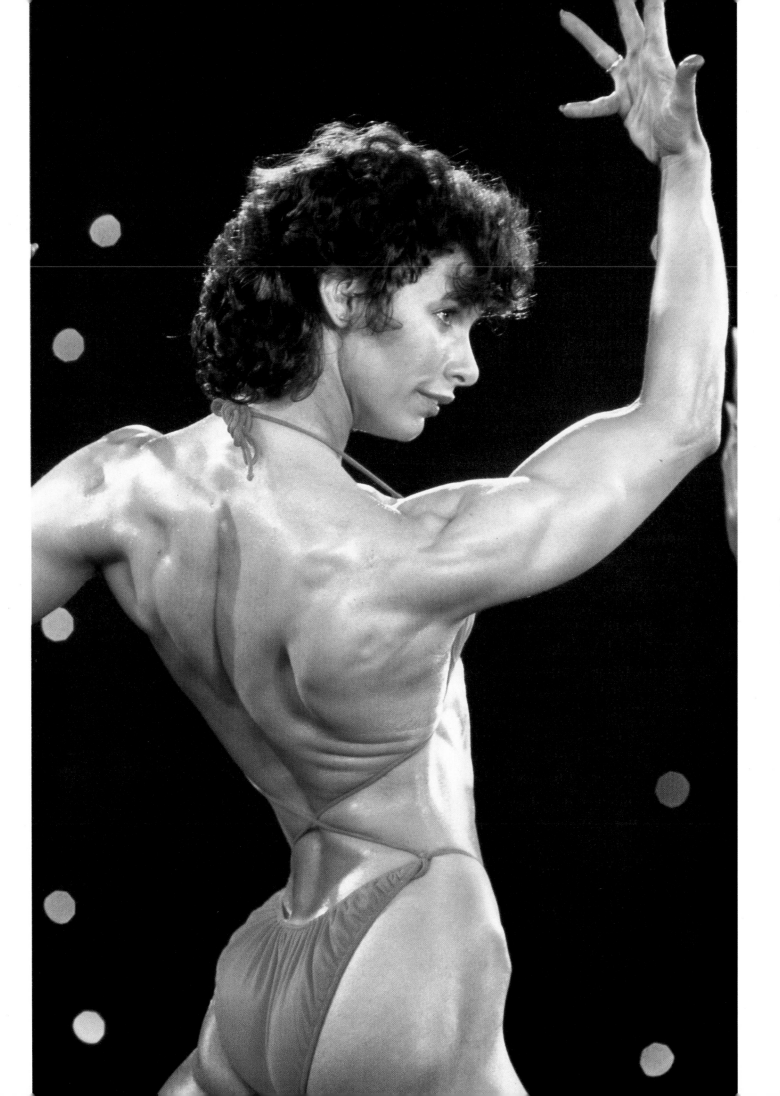

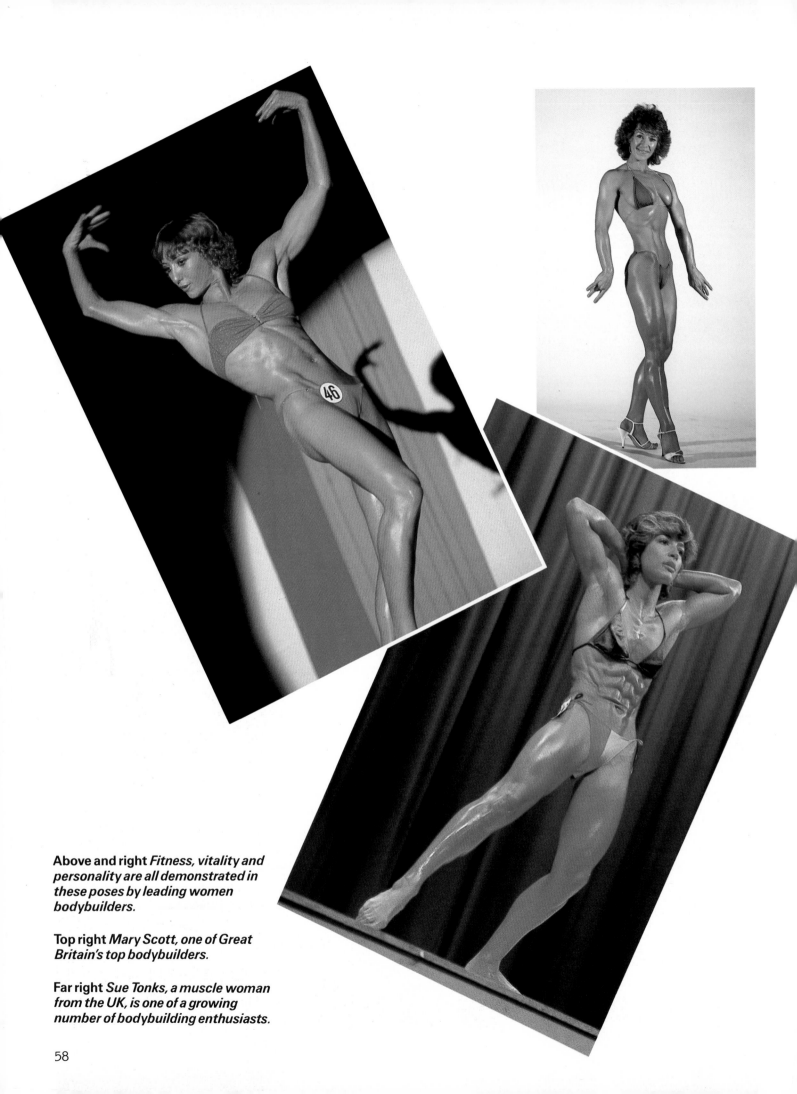

Above and right *Fitness, vitality and personality are all demonstrated in these poses by leading women bodybuilders.*

Top right *Mary Scott, one of Great Britain's top bodybuilders.*

Far right *Sue Tonks, a muscle woman from the UK, is one of a growing number of bodybuilding enthusiasts.*

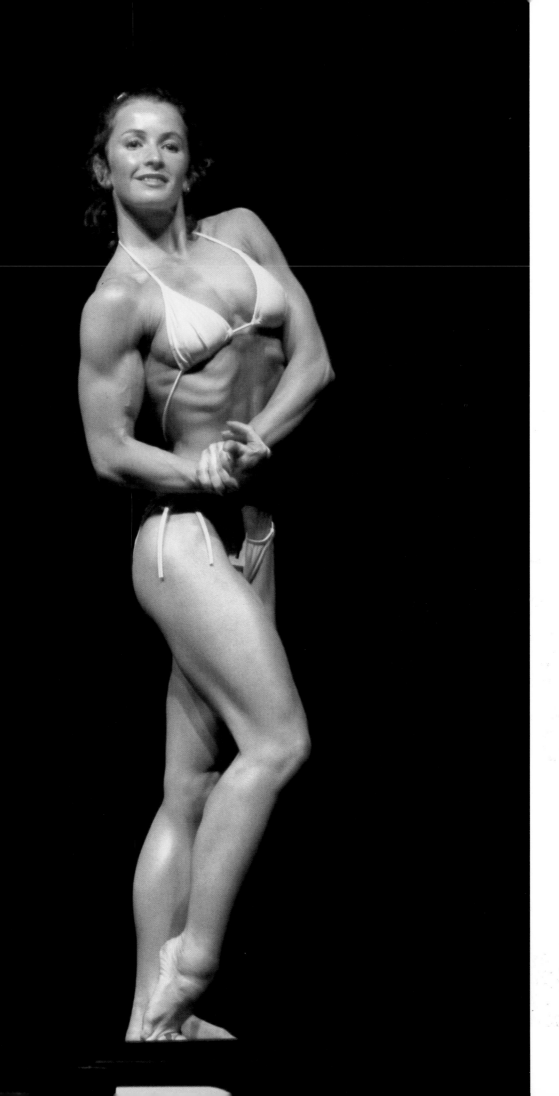

BASIC BODYBUILDING WITH WEIGHTS

The last section contained a program of freestanding exercises to loosen up and get fit, if you are taking your first steps in progressive training or any training for years. Many women prefer just to stick to the freestanding exercises to keep fit, but if you want to make your programs more interesting and show quick results, then you should get on to the bodybuilding exercises with weights. Below is a full list of all the exercises illustrated in Section II.

Warm up for three or four minutes on the gym bicycle. Then do one set of repetitions of arms circling, sidebends and trunk forward bends as illustrated in the freestanding program.

Then perform one set of alternate dumbell press. (One 'set' is completed when you repeat the exercise say 8 or 10 times. After a short breather, repeat the exercise again, with the same number of repetitions. You have now completed two 'sets'.) Progress to two sets of repetitions after about a month or so, unless you are pretty fit when you start. Two 5 to 10 lb dumbells should be heavy enough for a start.

Pick a chest and bust exercise next — such as the bench press. Again try one set, and progress to two sets, completing the two sets before you move to another exercise. Start at about 30 to 40 lbs.

The leg extension machine should come next, for the legs and thighs. But if you do not have access to a leg extension machine, try the squat with barbell (deep knee bend). Again, try two sets of repetitions after a month or so.

For the squat, try about 40 lbs — lighter for leg extensions, say 30 lbs.

Follow with straight arm pullover to restore breathing, improve rib cage, and so posture. Just a bar, about 15 to 20 lbs, is enough. Again, try one set, but in a month or so try two sets or repetitions.

For the mid-section use lying knees raise to chest from your freestanding program. One set at first, two later on.

Then do some hyperextensions as described in your freestanding program. Finally, assume the relaxation position.

This first bodybuilding program — combining freestanding exercises and weights — should take you about one hour, which is quite enough for one session.

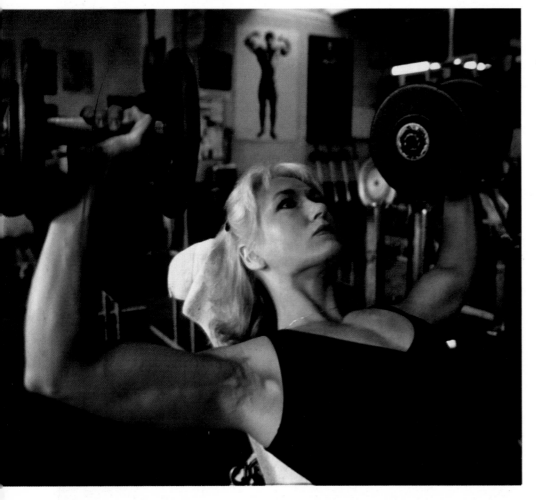

Left *Dumbell flying is a wonderful chest exercise.*

Right *A side chest pose shows upper body development.*

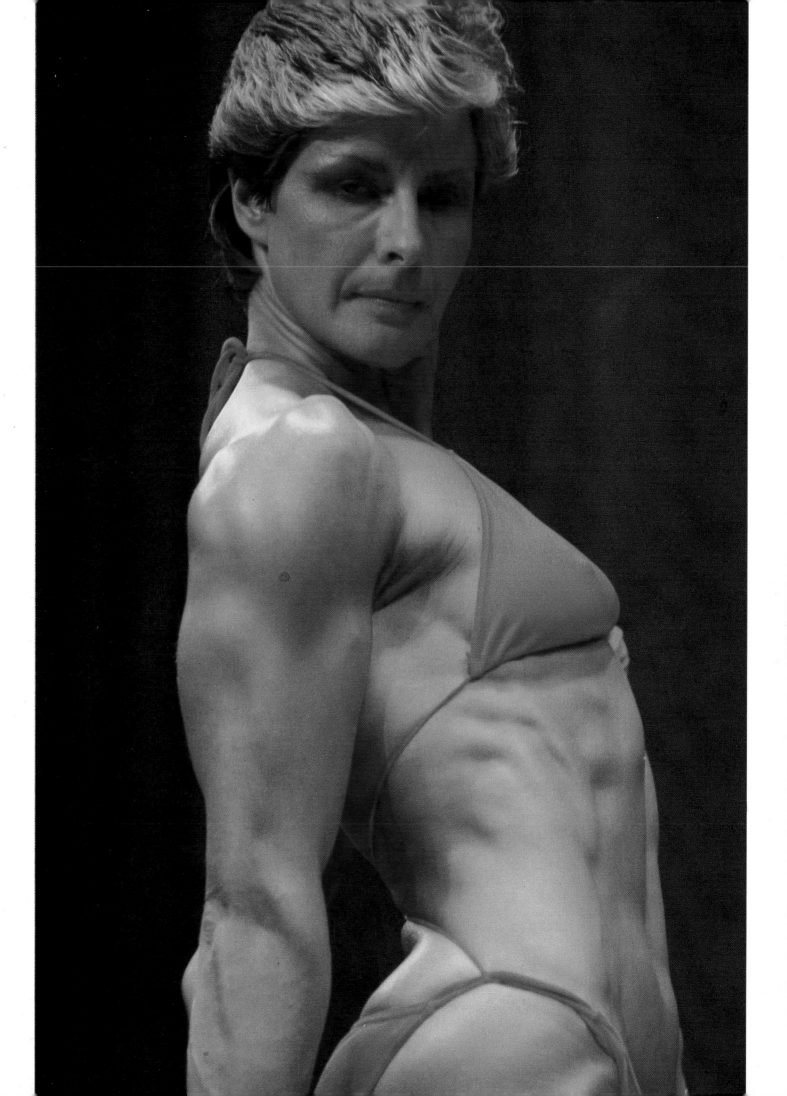

The clean

It is most important that you learn to pick up a barbell correctly from the floor to the shoulders. This is the commencing position of many of the exercises, and is also a fine back and leg exercise. The action of lifting the loaded barbell from the floor to the chest is called *the clean*. If you train at a club, you will be able to take the barbell off the stands, but taking the weight from the floor is a very good exercise in itself.

Stand with your legs slightly astride, feet about 15 ins apart, insteps against the barbell, toes pointing to the front. Bend your knees, keeping your back quite flat, hold your head and chest well up, and look straight ahead. Grasp the bar with both hands overgrip. The hands should be slightly more than shoulder-width apart. In this initial position with knees bent and seat near the floor, your arms must be kept straight with your heels flat on the floor.

Sink back on your heels and with a vigorous pull of the arms pull the bar upwards towards your chest. When the bar is as high as possible, twist your wrists quickly and pull the bar into the chest position, holding it high against your neck. Your elbows must be kept well up, with the weight resting mostly on the ball of the thumbs.

The lift must be done fast and in one continuous movement. It calls for speed and coordination, and may need practice. Breathe in just as you start the pull, and out as the bar reaches your chest.

Standing press with barbell

Stand with your feet astride and 'clean' the bar to your chest. Press the bar overhead keeping it as near to your face and body as possible. Do not look at the bar but straight ahead. Reach up as high as possible until your arms are in a straight line with your shoulders, above your head. There must be no body movement or jerking the bar overhead. Apart from a fine shoulder exercise, this is very good for faulty posture.

As a modest start try lifting 20 to 25 lbs. Try eight repetitions.

Alternate dumbell press

Pick up a pair of light dumbells, 8 to 10 lbs in weight. With dumbells parallel, pull them up to your shoulders. Hold them overgrasp with the thumbs round and the dumbells held high up at your shoulders and parallel. Without moving your lower body, press one dumbell overhead, keeping it near your head and past your ears. When one is on the way down the other goes up, in a continuous alternate movement. Keep your legs apart as in the previous exercise.

Breathe in normally as each dumbell travels upwards, and out as it comes back to your shoulders. Try alternate press to a count of 12.

Upright rowing

Stand with your feet about 15 ins apart. Hold the bar at the hang position, with your arms straight and hands about 4 ins apart, knuckles to the front. Pull the bar upwards by bending your elbows and raising them as high as possible, finishing with the bar under your chin. Keep the bar as close to you as possible. Lower to starting position.

Breathe in on the upward pull, and out as you lower the bar. Do eight to ten repetitions. Try about 20 lbs.

Pulley pull to back of neck

Pulleys form part of the regular equipment in any modern health studio. Sit facing the pulley. Grasp the bar with your hands about shoulder width apart (the pulley bars are quite long). Take a deep breath and pull the bar to the back of your neck, keeping firmly seated. Lean your head forward slightly to let the bar pass behind your neck. Let the bar touch the lower part of the back of the neck. Breathe in as you make the pull, and out as the bar returns to the upward starting position.

You should be able to manage 20 lbs or more, because it is not a difficult exercise.

Bench press with barbell

Lie on a flat bench, with your feet on either side and flat on the floor. With assistance, hold the bar at arms' length above your head, with hands slightly wider than shoulder width apart. Lower the bar to your chest under control until it touches your chest, then immediately press it off your chest to arms' length. Breathe in as the bar touches your chest, and out as you complete the press to arms' length. Try 35 lbs.

This exercise in some form is one of the best known of all bodybuilding exercises. It appears in all training programs both for men and women. It is also satisfying, because once you get used to it, you can make very rapid progress and increase the weight dramatically.

Bench press on machine

Most health studios now have a machine that can be used for this exercise. It has an advantage over the barbell bench press because you need no one to hand you the weight, and the poundages can be changed just by moving a pin up or down.

Lie on the bench as in the previous exercise. Grasp the bar across your chest and press it overhead. Breathing is as for the bench press with barbell. Breathe in as you commence the press, out as you return to the starting position. You can try possibly 10 more lbs than with a barbell.

Flying with dumbells

Lie on a bench with your feet on either side and flat on the floor. Hold a dumbell at arms' length in each hand, dumbells parallel. Lower the dumbell outwards by bending your arms, until they are below chest level. As you get used to the exercise, lower them wide, but not with arms straight. Return to the overhead starting position and repeat. Breathe in as the dumbells are lowered outwards, and out as you return to the starting position. 5 lb dumbells are enough to start with because this is a hard exercise if done correctly.

Pec deck machine

This is a fairly new type of machine, but it is an excellent one for contracting the chest muscles. Sit at the machine and grasp the levers that are outwards, with your forearms against the padded part. Pull the two levers together until they meet almost in front of you. Breathe in as you make the pull, and out as you return to the starting position. Repeat 8 to 10 times. You can try a little more weight with these than with the dumbells — about 10 to 15 lbs.

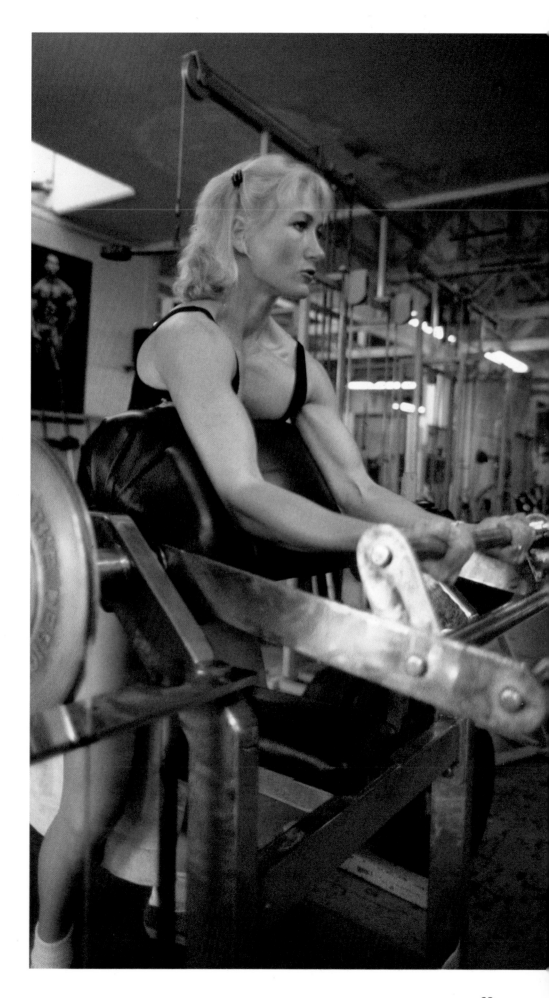

Curls are one of the many basic exercises used for developing the upper arms.

Straight arm pullover

This is primarily a shoulder and upper back exercise, but it has a marked effect on the rib box and posture. The exercise is most often used after squats or knees bend, to restore the breathing back to normal.

Lie on a bench, with your feet on either side of it and flat on the floor. Hold a bar at arms' length about your head. Your grip should be slightly wider than shoulder width. Keep your arms almost straight, although a slight bend in the elbows is advisable if you are a little tight in the shoulders. Lower the bar behind your head, until it is in line with your shoulders, so that arms and body are in a straight line. Pull the bar back, but continue the movement to the thighs, completing a 180° movement with the bar. Breathe very deeply as the bar goes backwards behind your head, and out all the way back. Be sure that there is no hip lift off the bench.

This is a great exercise for the respiratory system, mobilizing the whole of the rib cage.

Squat (knees bend)

This is an exercise for thighs and back, and also a great stamina-builder, because it has a very marked effect on breathing. It should be included in some form in every training program for sportspeople. Stand with your feet astride about 15 ins, with a bar across your shoulders. In most health clubs there are racks to take the bar from, but if not, you will need assistance to put the bar behind your head. Toes must point to the front, and unless you can keep your heels flat on the floor when you commence the knees bend, you must put a block of wood or something similar about 2 to 4 ins high under your heels. Many people find this necessary. Take a deep breath and, keeping your back flat, bend your knees until your thighs are parallel with the floor. Make sure that you do not squat too far and sag, because it might produce lower back strain. As soon as you think that your thighs are parallel to the floor, return to the standing position.

Breathe in when you make your effort, so supplying the necessary oxygen for the blood. The effort in this case takes place as you come up from the squat position. It would be very difficult to take a deep breath in this position, so breathe in deeply just before you commence the knees bend, and out as you return to the standing position.

You can try about 40 lbs. You may find it easy to increase the poundages

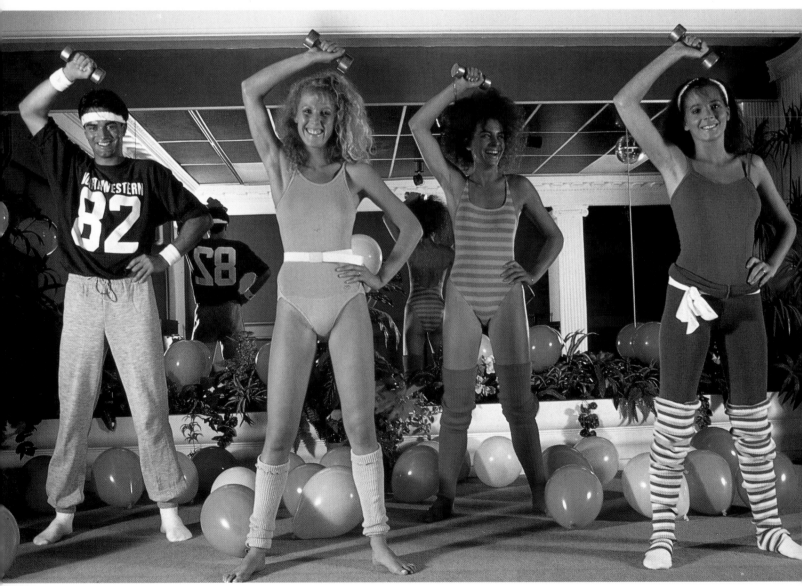

in this exercise, but you should preferably use light weights and high repetitions for shaping the thighs and shedding the odd inch or two. Heavy squats may enlarge your hips and bottom.

Leg extensions

The leg extension machine is found in all modern health clubs. This is not quite an alternative to squats but it is very good for tightening up the thighs, for minor knee injuries, and for strengthening the area round the knees. As a result, it is ideal for athletic persons.

Sit at the machine and tuck your instep under the bar. Hold the bench part, unless handles are provided. Without any body movement but by contracting the thigh muscles, raise the bar until your legs are at right angles to your body. Lower and repeat 8 to 10 times. Breathe in as you straighten your legs, and out as you lower the bar. This machine is adjustable with a pin. Try about 20 to 30 lbs. You can also reverse the machine for the backs of the thighs.

Calf machine

If you have access to a calf machine, do use it. These machines are simple to use and molding the calf, even if it looks slim, is as important as treating the thighs.

Sidebends with barbell

Stand astride with your feet about 15 ins apart and toes pointing to the front. With just a bar (about 16 lbs) balanced on your shoulders and keeping the body square to the front, bend from side to side, as far to each side as possible, to a count of 16 to 20. Breathe freely. This is very good for that 'spare tire'.

Sidebends with dumbells

This is the same as sidebends with barbell, but less restricted, because you can move your head freely, so giving your neck some exercise. Both sidebend exercises are really very similar.

Sit-ups on abdominal board

Most health clubs have abdominal boards, and they are useful if only because you do not need the assistance of somebody to hold your feet. They are made so that you can adjust the angle of sitting up. If you want to use one at first, use a flat board. When you start raising the board, never go beyond a 45° angle, otherwise the exercise becomes a thigh exercise, instead of one for the abdomen.

Continue with the lying knees raise and legs raise as you progress.

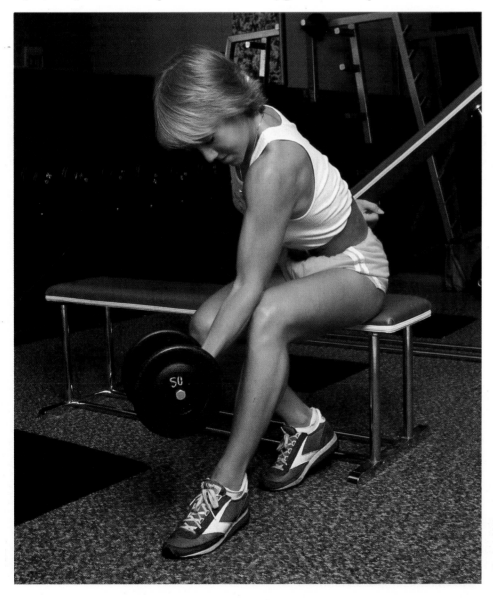

Far left *Bodybuilding and aerobics can prove a fun combination.*

Left *The seated dumbell curl helps develop the arms.*

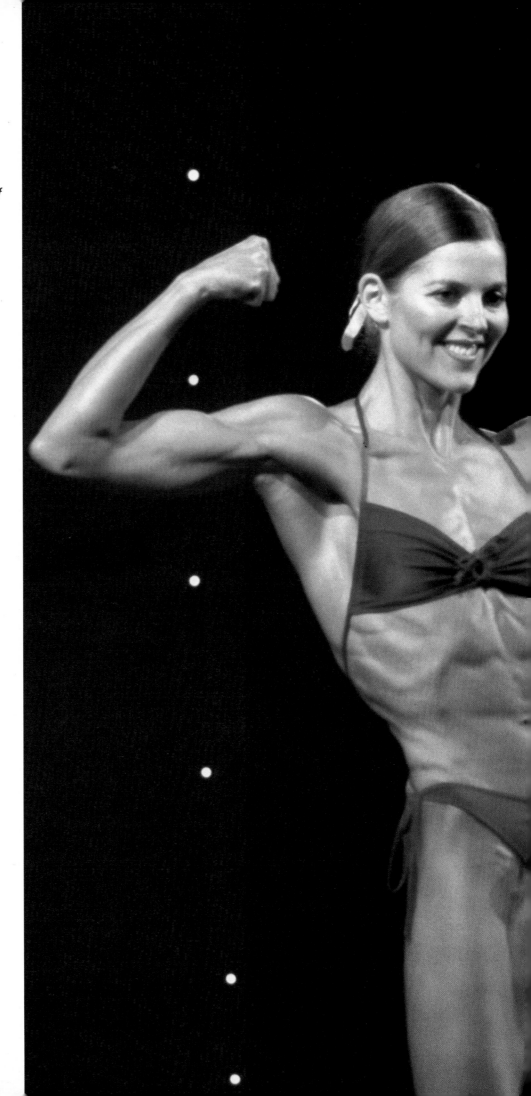

British bodybuilders Angelito Lesta and Carolyn Cheshire regularly compete in competitions worldwide.

Inset *Carolyn Cheshire of the UK displays her muscular upper arms. Muscularity like this can be yours — if that's what you want.*

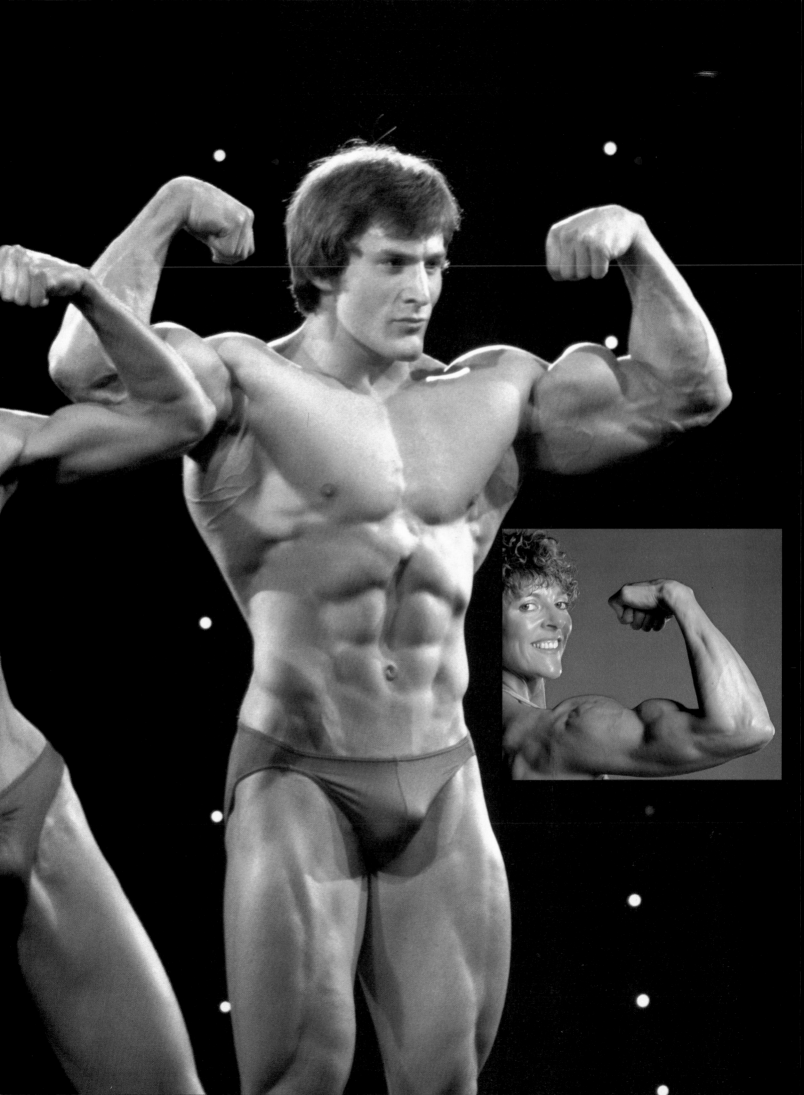

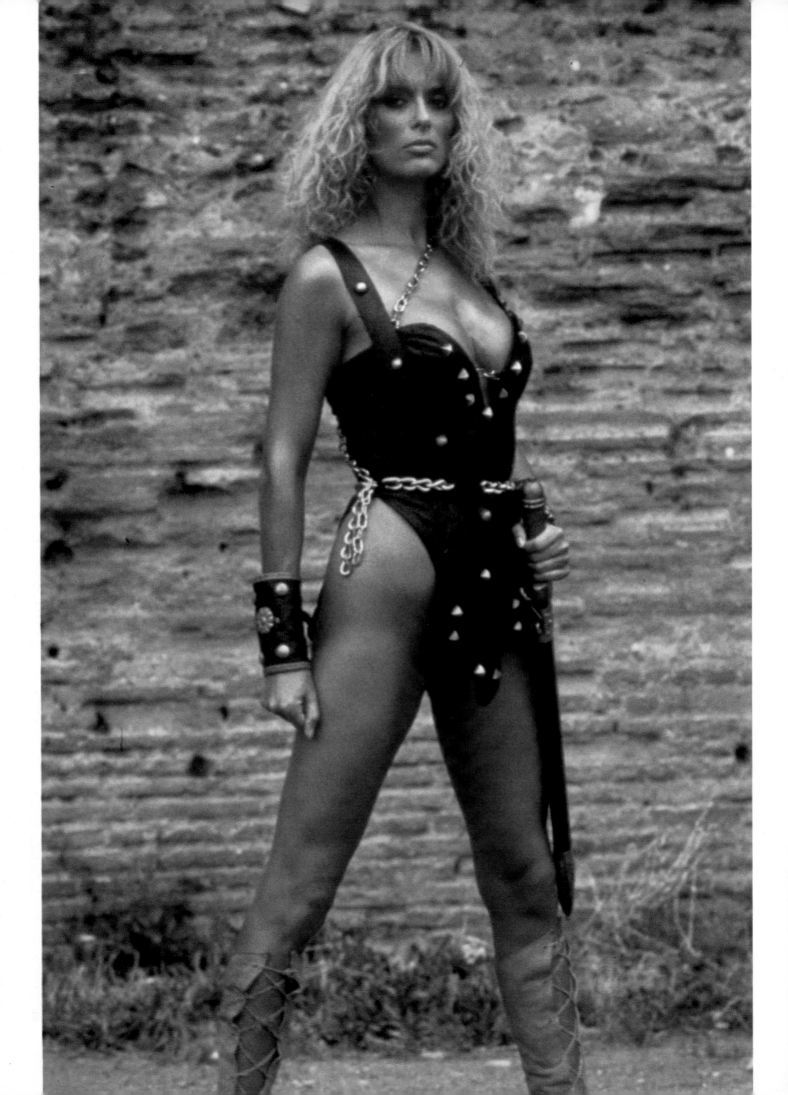

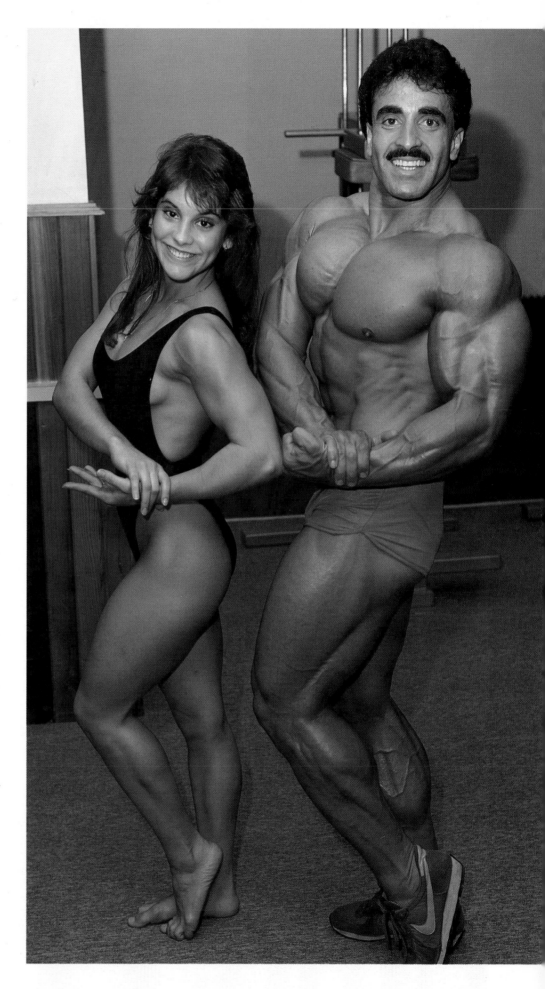

Left *Fit and ready for glamorous action.*

Right *One of the world's top men bodybuilders, Samir Bannout, poses with an up-and-coming girl.*

Following pages *Bodybuilding 'gadgets' can be effective — if combined with a regular workout program.*

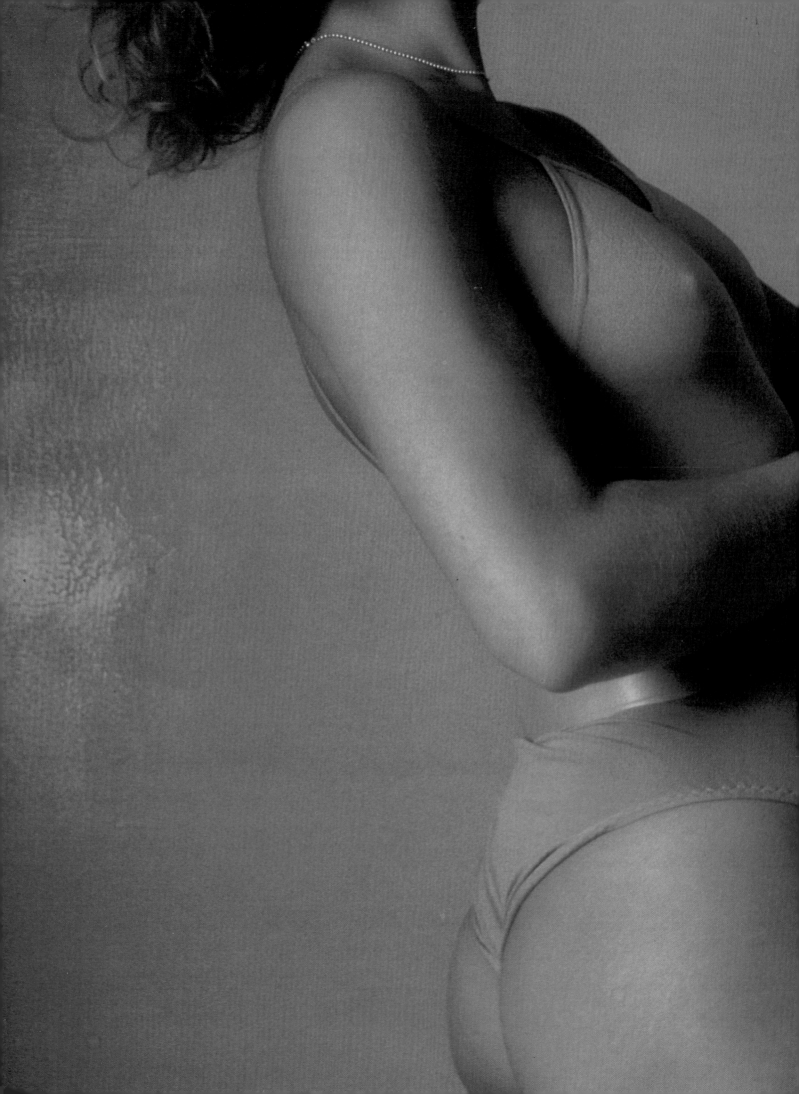

THE IDEAL WORKOUT PROGRAM

After an initial period — depending on your progress and how often you can work out — your program should look something like this:

Warm up on the gym bicycle for three or four minutes. Spend another five minutes on some bending and stretching from your freestanding exercises. Then do the following:

Press with barbell   2 sets of 10 repetitions. Complete the two sets before going on to the next exercise. 25 lbs.

Upright rowing   2 sets of 10 repetitions. Complete the two sets before going on to the next exercise. 20 lbs.

Squat with barbell   2 sets of 10 repetitions. Complete 2 sets before going to the next exercise. 50 lbs.

Straight arm pullover with barbell   1 set of 15 repetitions full movement. 15 to 18 lbs.

Bench press   2 sets of 10 repetitions. Complete 2 sets before going to the next exercise. 40 lbs.

Pec deck   1 set of 10 repetitions. 30 lbs.

Sidebends with bar across shoulders   1 set of 16 repetitions.

Lying sit-ups   2 sets of 8 repetitions, or use an abdominal board.

Standing side kicks   Repeat 16 times, 8 with each leg.

Hyperextensions   10 repetitions.

Relaxation and breathing.

Do not have long breaks between sets of exercises. The break should be not more than three or four minutes in order to get your breathing back to normal and to relax before the next effort. A little self-discipline is often needed here because once you lose concentration and continuity you may as well retire to the sauna.

SECTION II
COLOR GUIDE TO BODYBUILDING EXERCISES

*The exercises illustrated and described in this section
are the basic exercises that are most popular for beginners
of any age of natural ability. The models used are
young people who have been training for one or two years —
just to keep fit and healthy.
They work on the exercises described in these pages
for approximately one hour three times a week.
So good luck — and good training!*

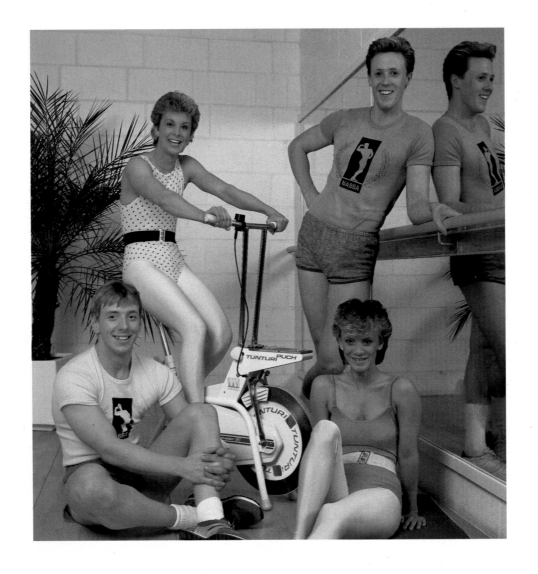

Exercise bicycles are standard equipment in most exercise centers and are also popular for home use. An excellent way to warm up before your training program, the bicycle also exercises the legs and improves the respiration.
Be modest and start with light resistance for two or three minutes.

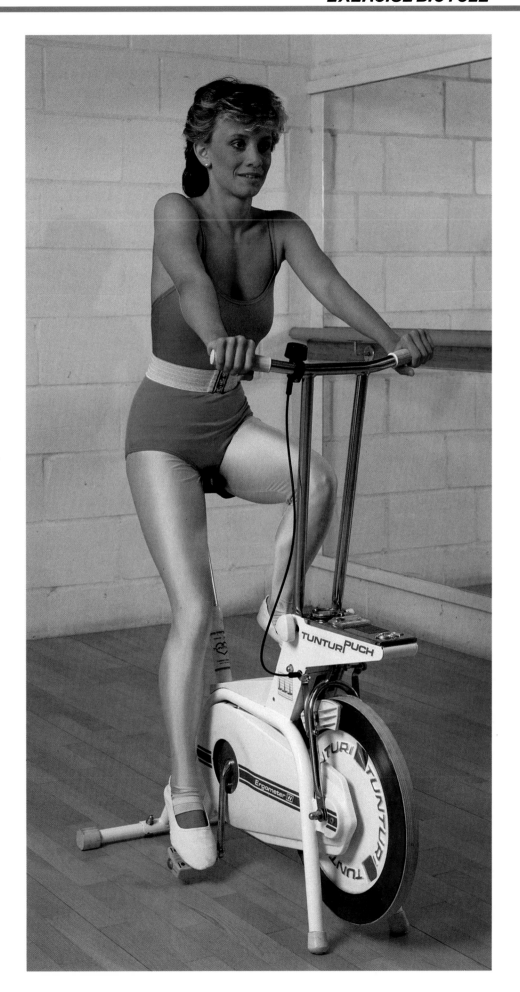

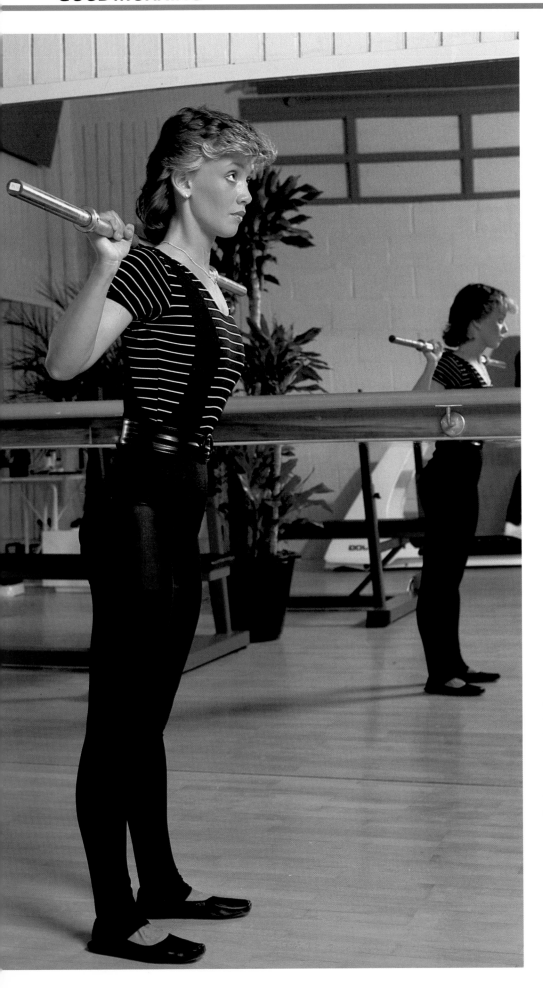

Stand feet astride, a very light bar across your shoulders behind your neck. Keep the head well up (left). If you are out of condition, bend your knees when doing this exercise. Bend forward until the body is at right angles to the legs, forcing your head back so that the bar does not lose position (right).
In time try and go further down towards your knees, but only when you are really fit and supple.
Breathing: Inhale just as you commence the forward bend; exhale as you return to the upright.
This exercise gives the back and the backs of the legs a good stretch, but care must be taken if you have any sort of back injury.

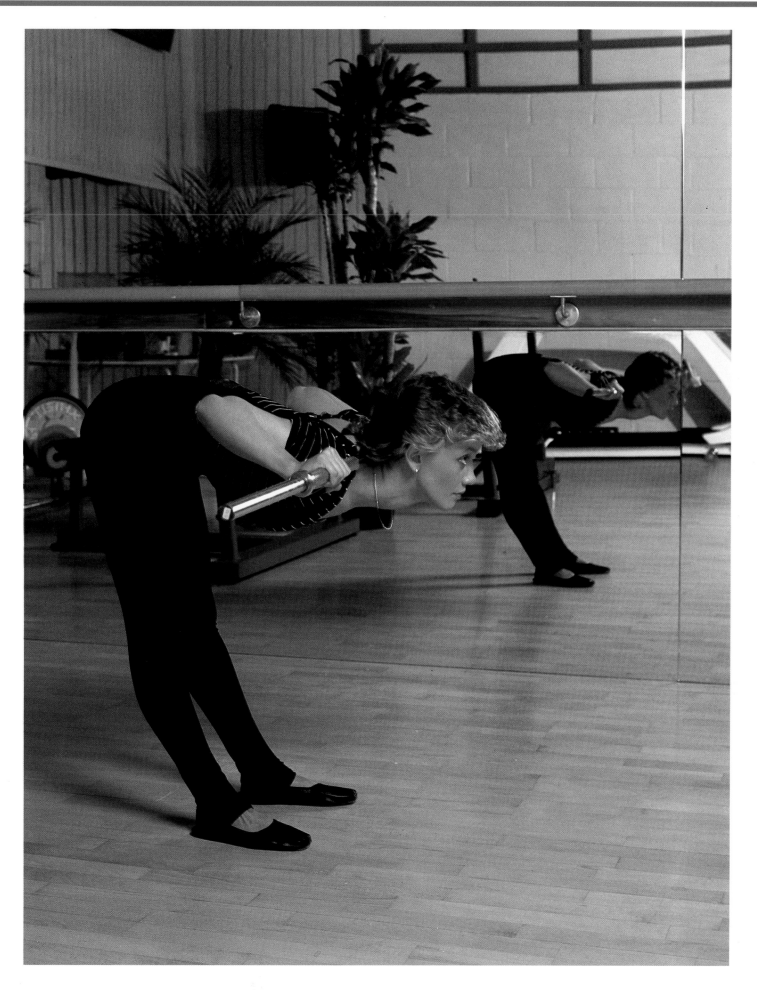

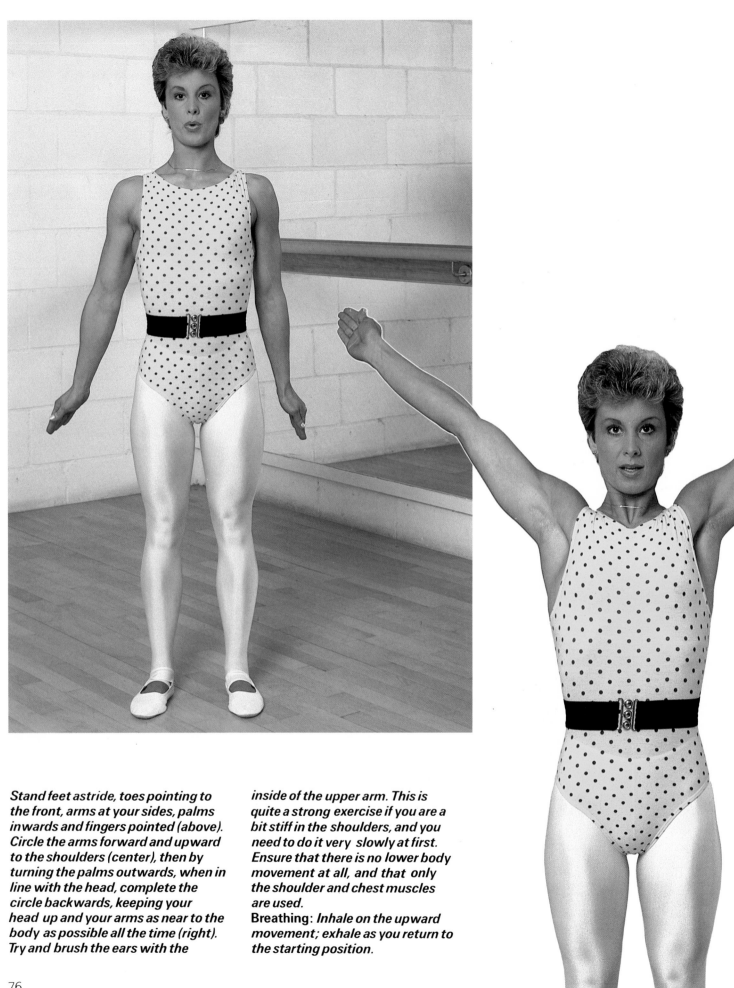

Stand feet astride, toes pointing to the front, arms at your sides, palms inwards and fingers pointed (above). Circle the arms forward and upward to the shoulders (center), then by turning the palms outwards, when in line with the head, complete the circle backwards, keeping your head up and your arms as near to the body as possible all the time (right). Try and brush the ears with the inside of the upper arm. This is quite a strong exercise if you are a bit stiff in the shoulders, and you need to do it very slowly at first. Ensure that there is no lower body movement at all, and that only the shoulder and chest muscles are used.

Breathing: *Inhale on the upward movement; exhale as you return to the starting position.*

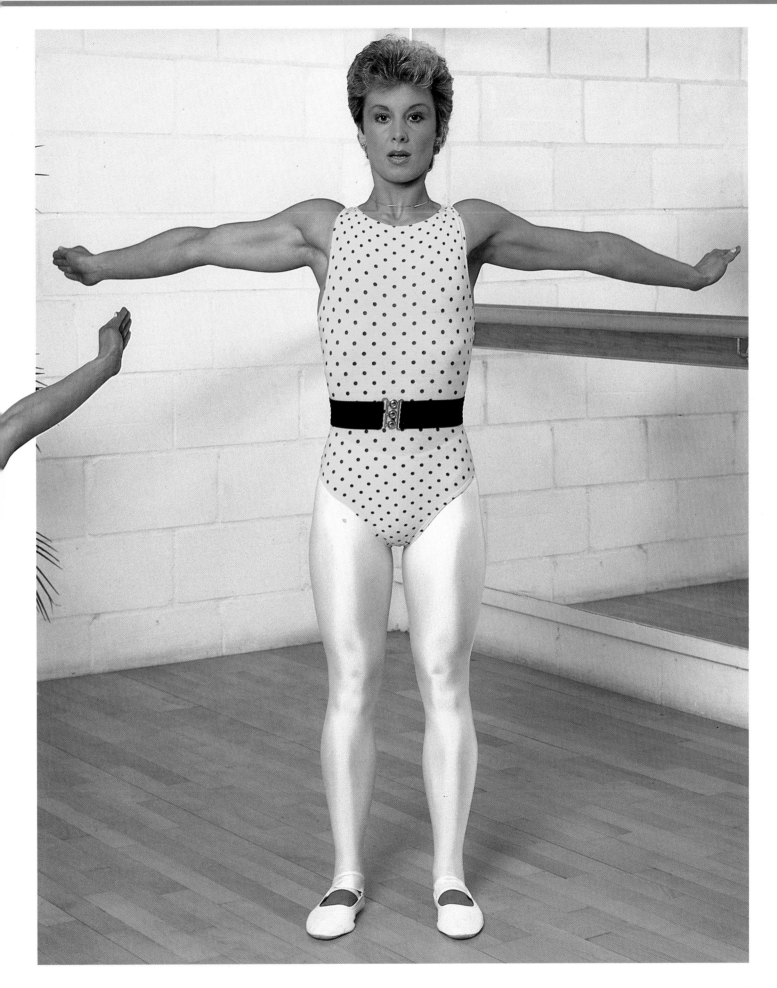

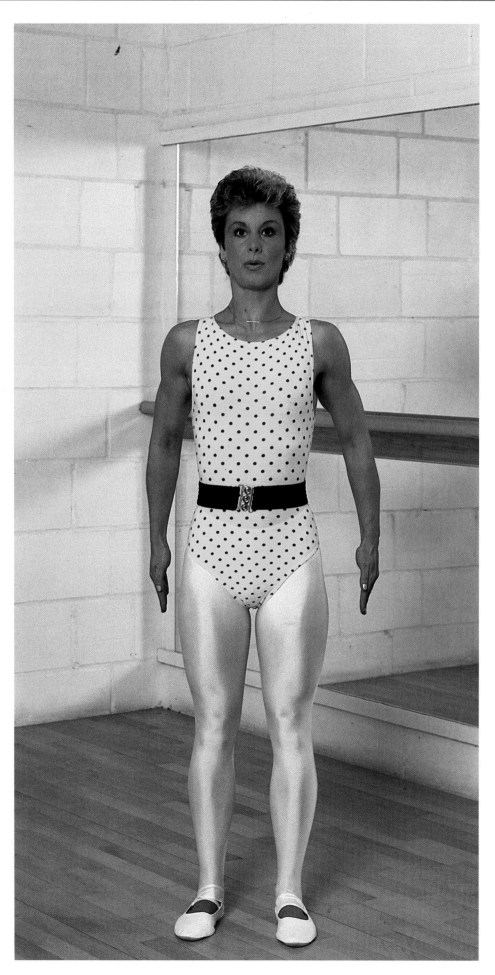

Stand feet not too wide astride, toes pointing to the front. Hands at sides, palms facing inwards (left).
Without any lower body movement at all or jerking, swing the arms, keeping them fairly close to the head, upwards, until the inside of your arms are approaching your ears (right).
If you are a little stiff in the shoulders you may find this difficult at first, but whatever you do, do not lean back to complete the movement. Look straight ahead and do not raise your heels off the floor.
Breathing: Inhale deeply on the upward movement; exhale as your arms come to starting position.
A fine exercise for posture.

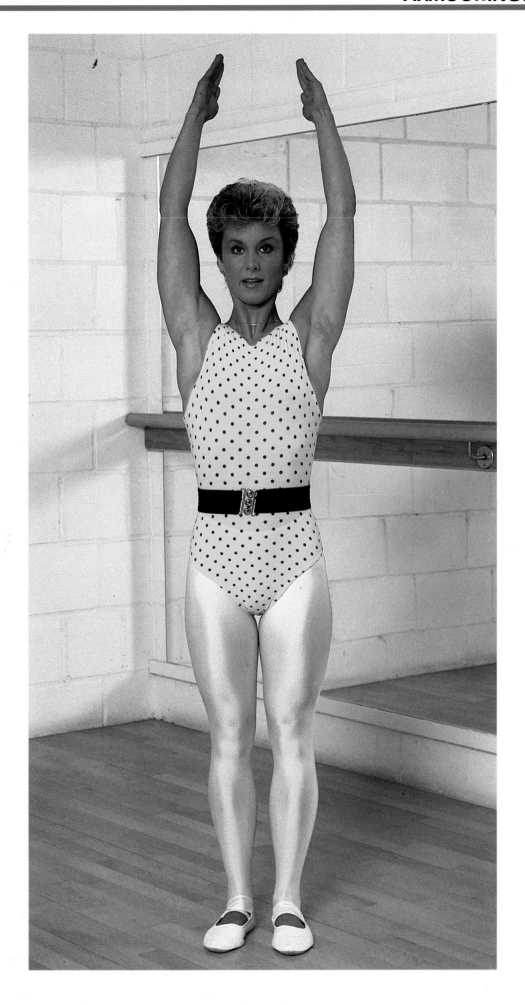

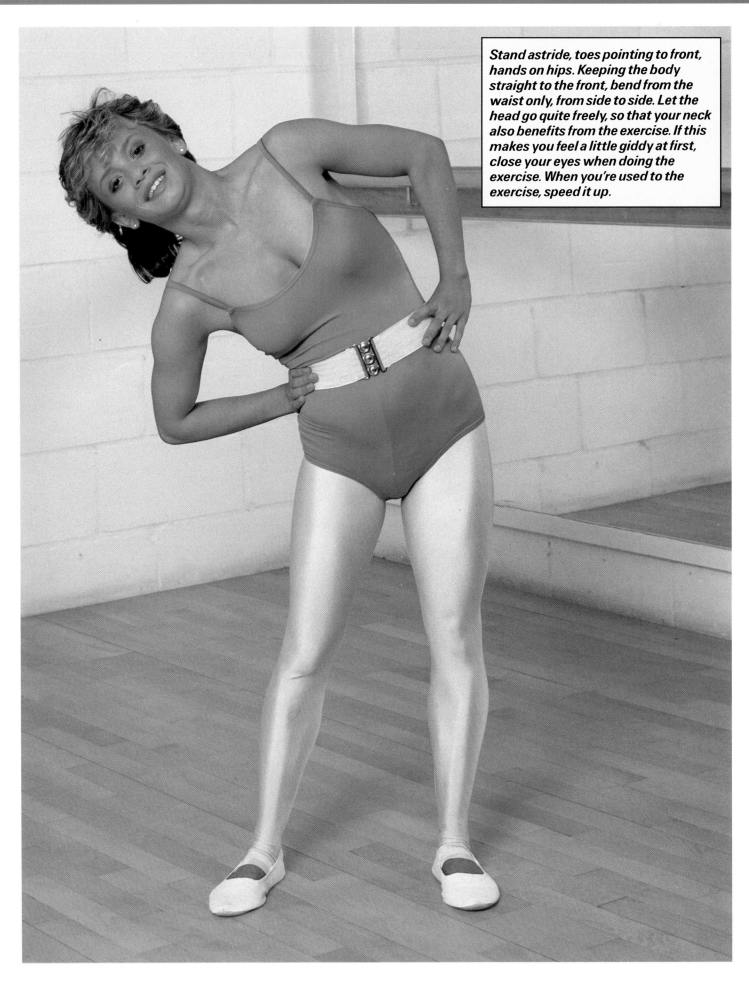

Stand astride, toes pointing to front, hands on hips. Keeping the body straight to the front, bend from the waist only, from side to side. Let the head go quite freely, so that your neck also benefits from the exercise. If this makes you feel a little giddy at first, close your eyes when doing the exercise. When you're used to the exercise, speed it up.

Your body may not move very far at first either to the left or right, but you should eventually get your upper body at right angles to your lower body.
Breathing: *Try and breathe quite freely.*
Great for the waist if done with high repetitions.

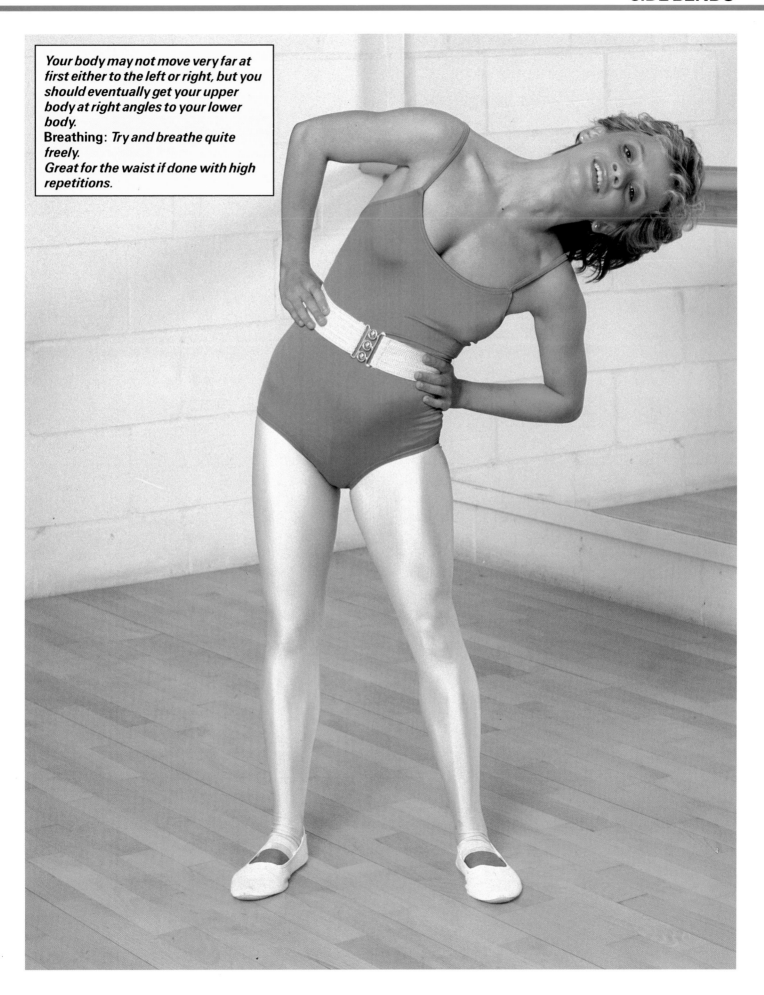

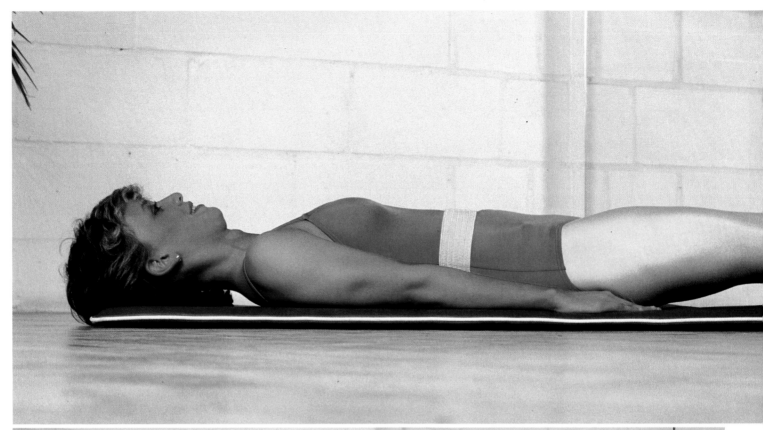

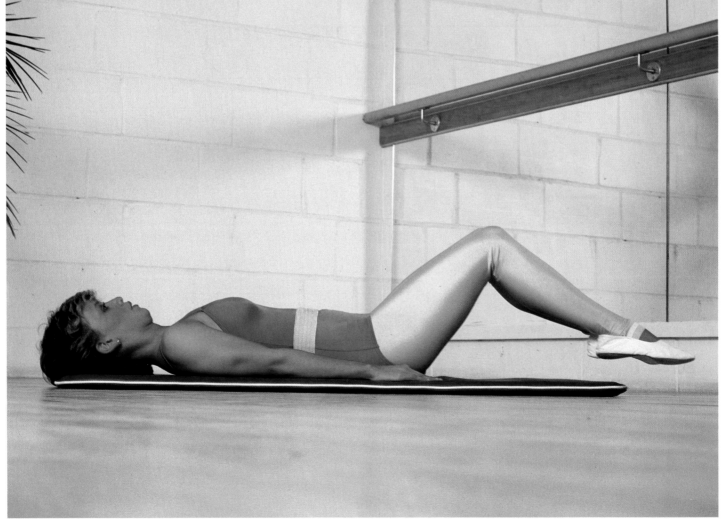

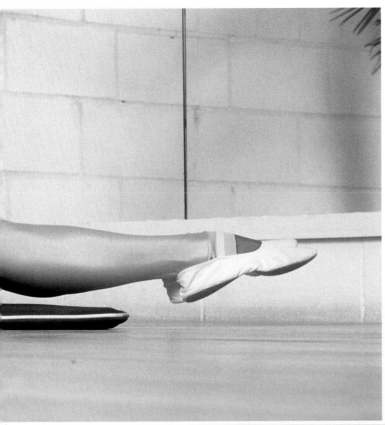

Lie on the floor, legs straight and toes pointed. Hands at the sides, palms of hands on the floor. Take a deep breath and raise both knees to the chest keeping them pressed tightly together. Return to starting position breathing out. Raise the knees as far as possible towards the chest.
Breathing: *Inhale when raising the knees; exhale when returning to the starting position.*
This is a strong exercise for the tummy muscles, so if you are weak, or not too young, try alternate knee raising.

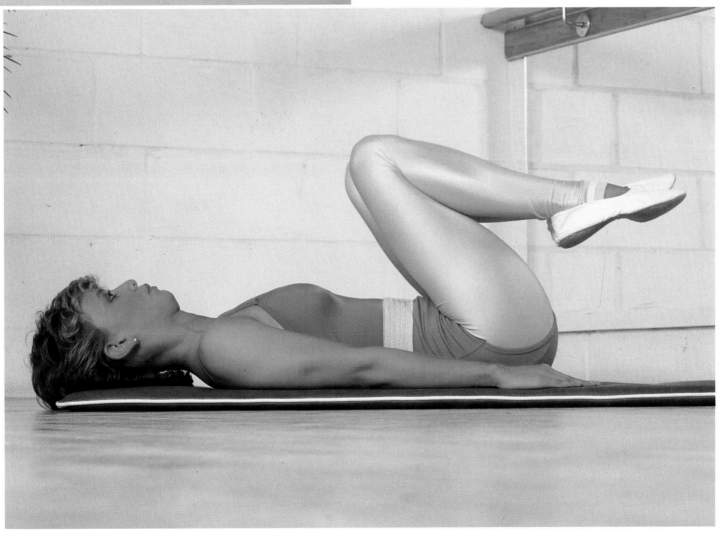

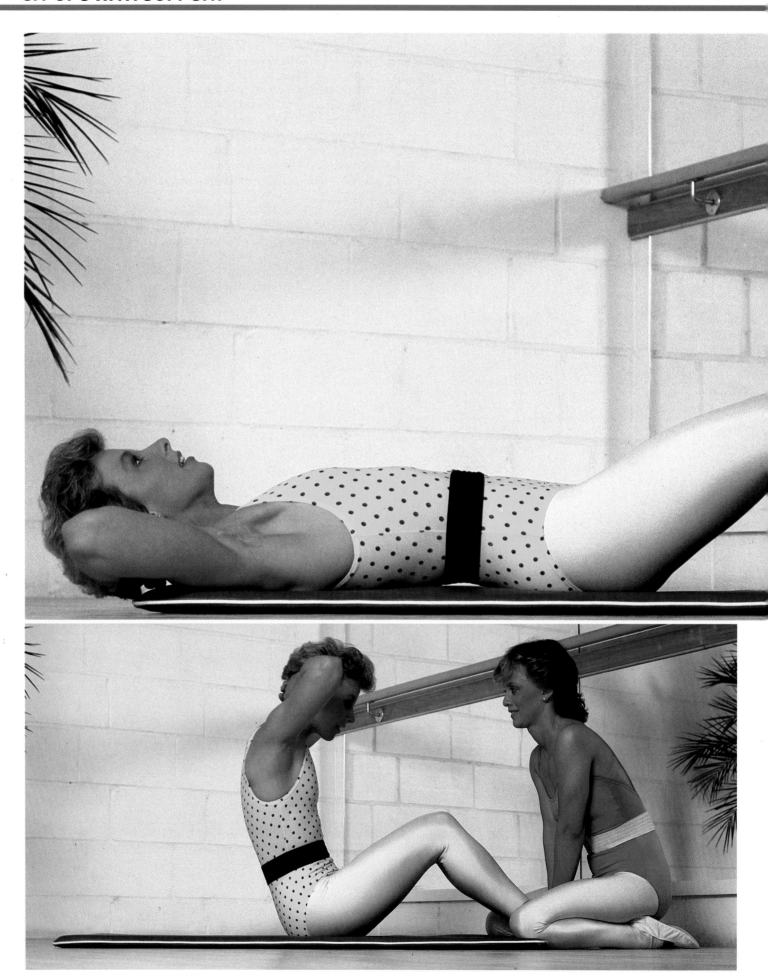

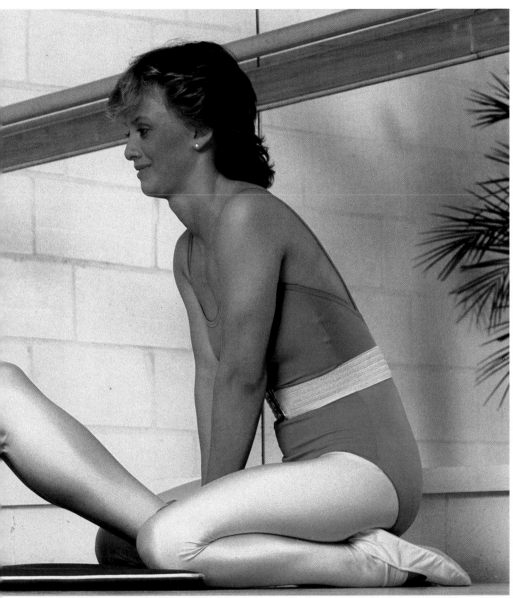

Lie on the floor, feet together, toes pointed, arms in the 'neck rest' position, knees slightly bent. Anchor your feet, or have the assistance of a partner. Swing the body forward and sit up, reaching forward as far as possible, and bending the body towards the thighs. This is a difficult exercise and fairly advanced. You can start by sitting and then just reaching toward the outstretched legs. When you can put your head flat on your insteps, then you have become really supple and strong in the tummy muscles.

Breathing: *Take a deep breath just as you swing the arms forward, and breathe out as you lie back.*

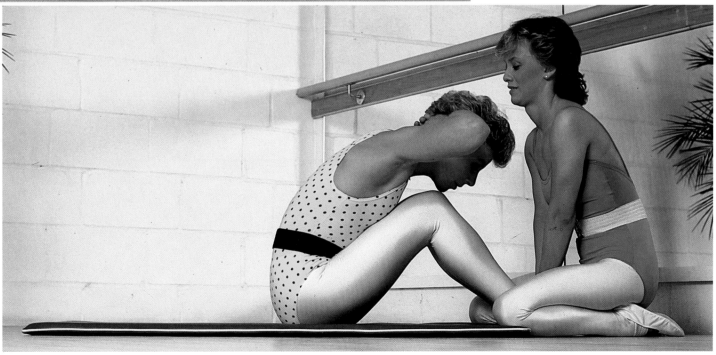

85

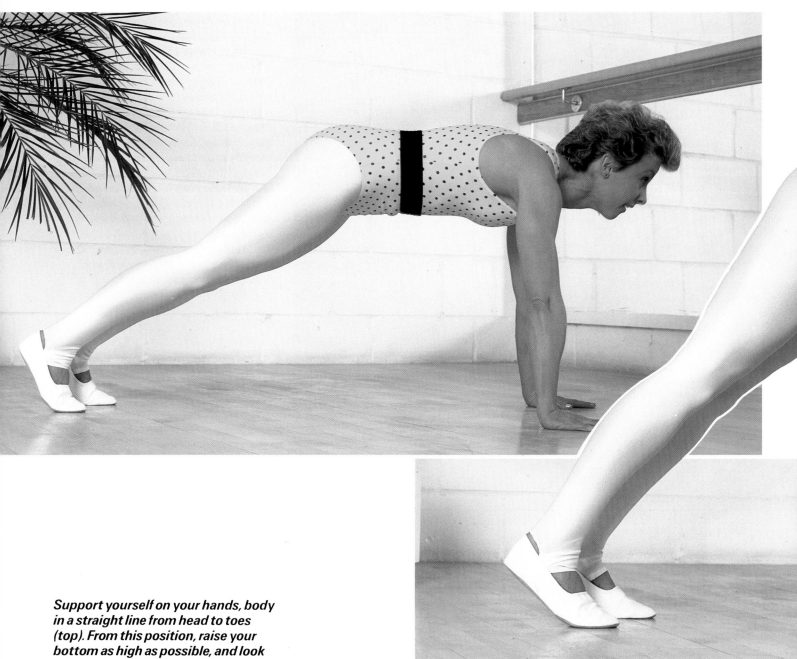

Support yourself on your hands, body in a straight line from head to toes (top). From this position, raise your bottom as high as possible, and look towards your feet, making an inverted 'V' shape (center).
Try and force your heels to the floor. From the 'V' position, without moving your hands, sag in the middle, until your hips touch the floor and force the head back (right). Return to the starting position and repeat several times. When in the arched position it is a good thing to try three or four times forcing your heels to the floor, and your head towards your knees. This is a hard exercise, but one for many muscle groups and great for making the back supple and the arms and tummy muscles stronger.
Breathing: *Inhale deeply as you arch the body; exhale as you sag towards the ground.*

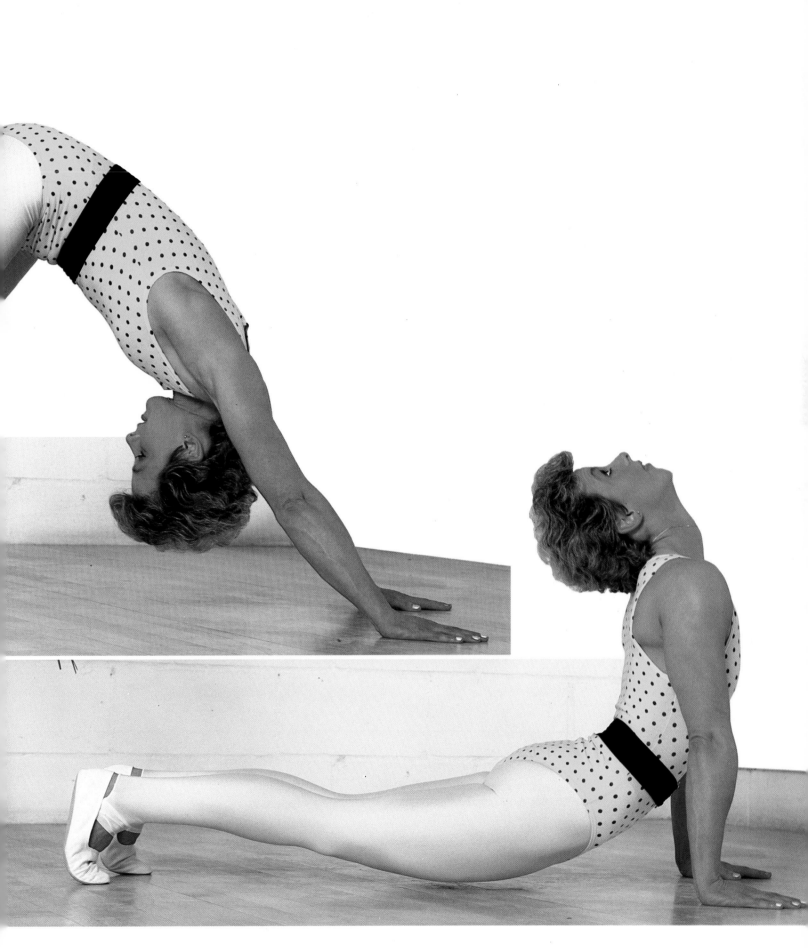

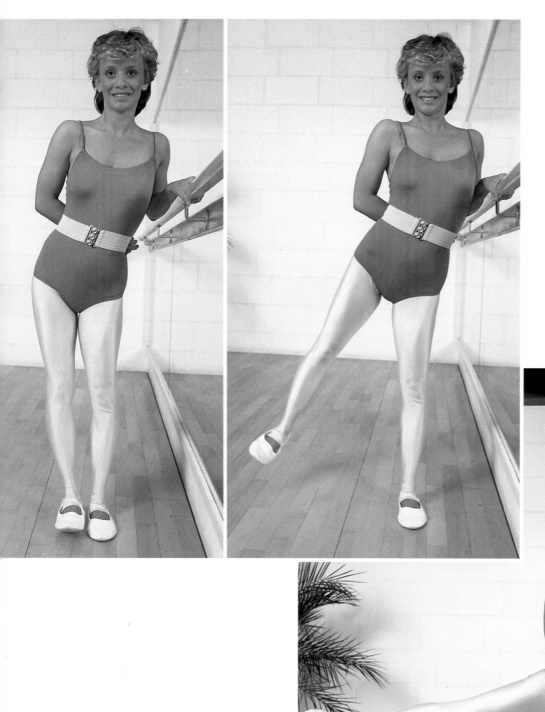

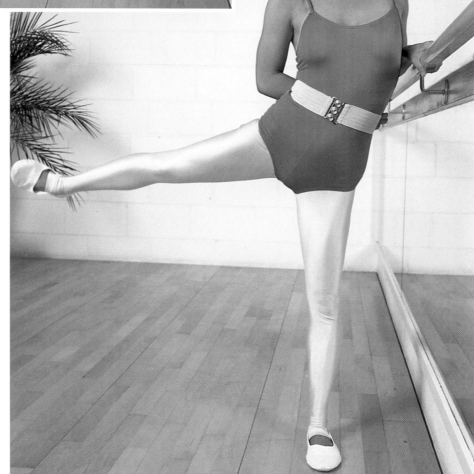

Many health clubs have a 'ballet bar' which is ideal for this exercise. Position yourself at the bar as shown in the illustrations. Point the toe and raise the leg as high as possible. Perform one set of repetitions with one leg, then repeat with the other.
Breathing: *Breathe normally.*
Very good for the inside muscles of the legs.

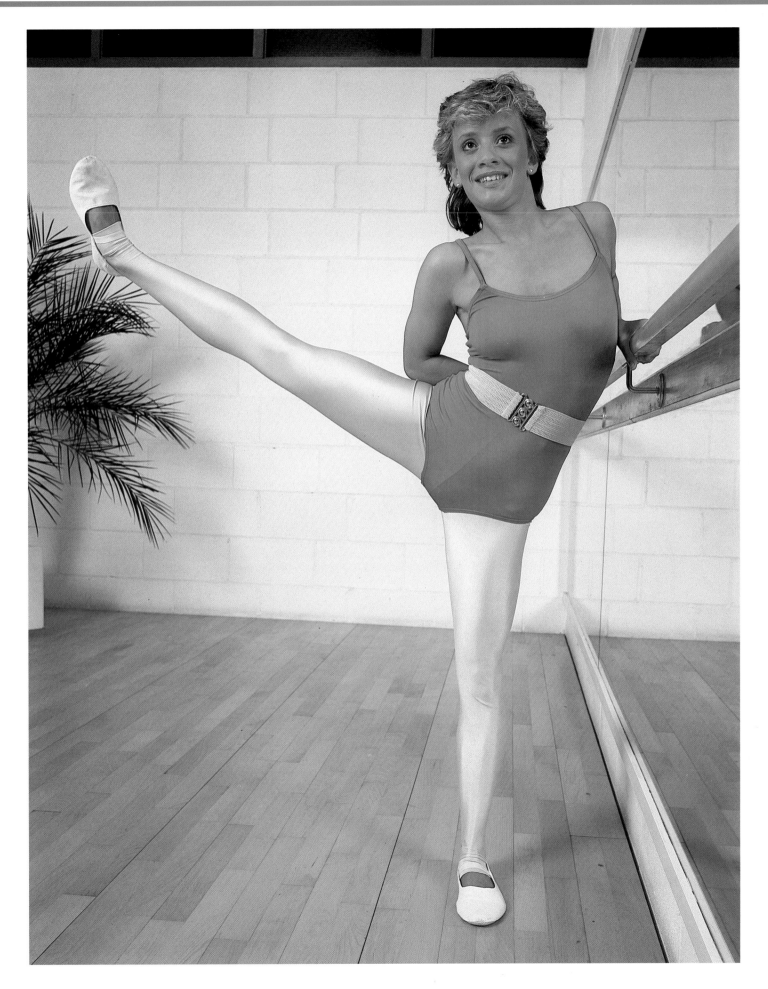

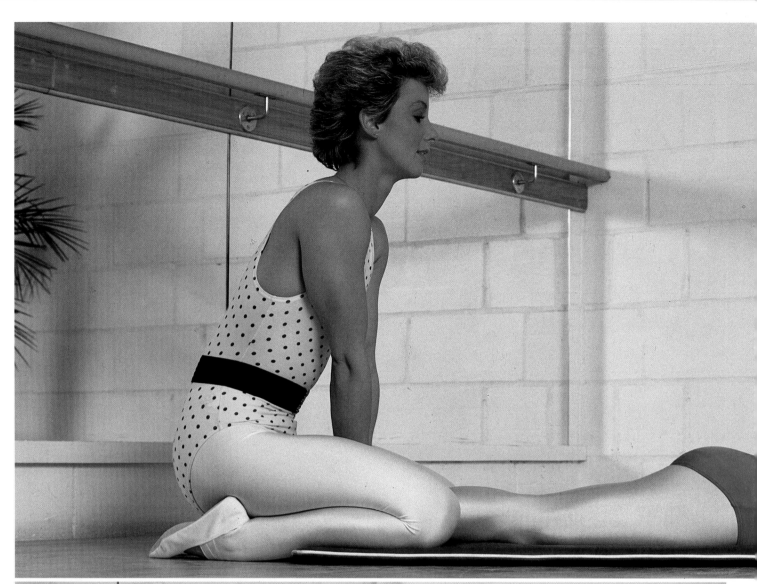

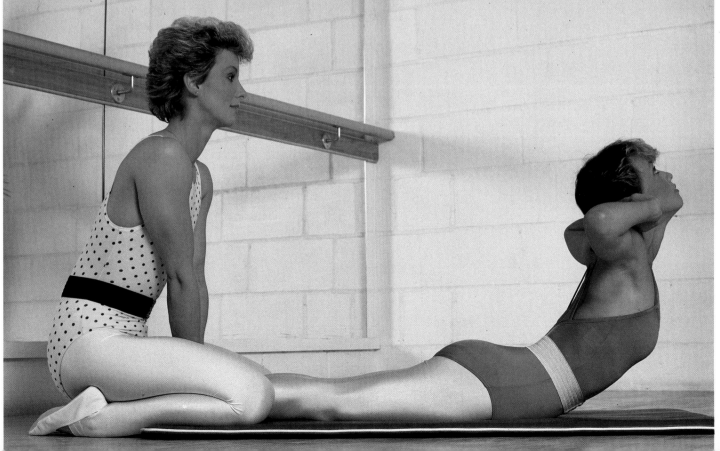

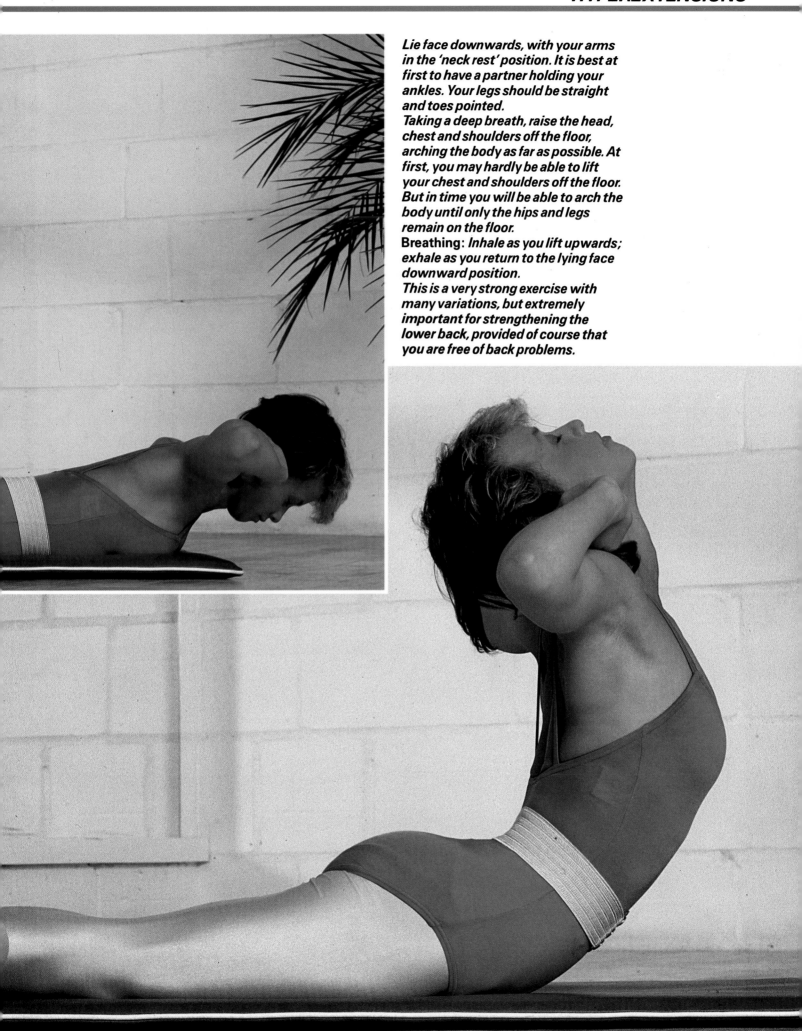

Lie face downwards, with your arms in the 'neck rest' position. It is best at first to have a partner holding your ankles. Your legs should be straight and toes pointed.

Taking a deep breath, raise the head, chest and shoulders off the floor, arching the body as far as possible. At first, you may hardly be able to lift your chest and shoulders off the floor. But in time you will be able to arch the body until only the hips and legs remain on the floor.

Breathing: *Inhale as you lift upwards; exhale as you return to the lying face downward position.*

This is a very strong exercise with many variations, but extremely important for strengthening the lower back, provided of course that you are free of back problems.

The clean

'Cleaning' a weight means picking a barbell or dumbells up from the floor to the shoulders in one continuous movement, using the back and leg muscles.

Stand legs astride, but not too apart, toes pointing to the front, insteps touching the bar if you are lifting a barbell (below). Bend the knees keeping the back quite flat, and holding the head and chest well up looking straight ahead of you. Grasp the bar overgrip, with the thumbs round the bar so there is no chance of your hands slipping. The hands should be slightly more than shoulder width apart, knuckles uppermost. With the knees bent and the thighs parallel to the floor, sink back on the heels, and with a vigorous pull of the arms, pull the bar to the chest in one continuous movement. When the bar is as high as possible towards the chin, twist the wrists quickly and pull the bar into position across the front of the chest and high up on the neck (opposite page). The weight of the bar is taken mostly on the ball part of the hands. Keep the elbows well up.
Breathing: *Inhale as you pull, and exhale as the bar reaches the neck and upper chest.*

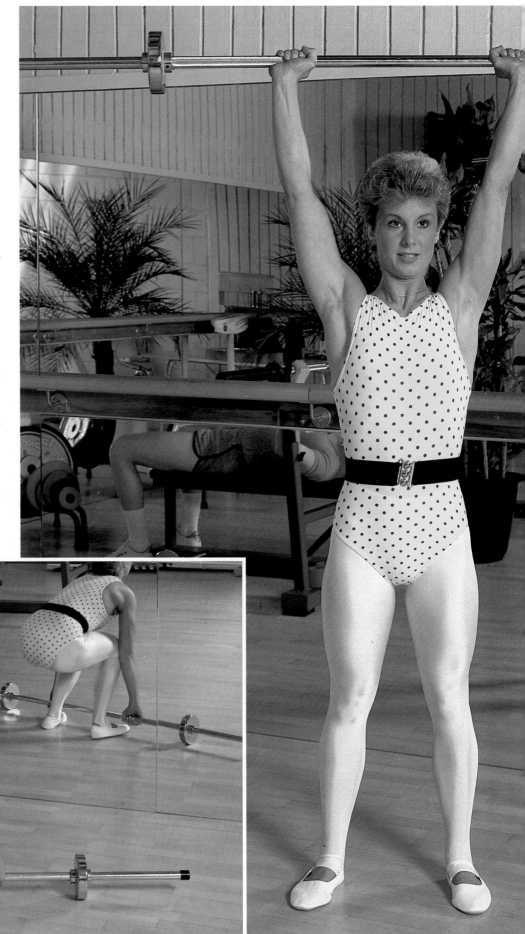

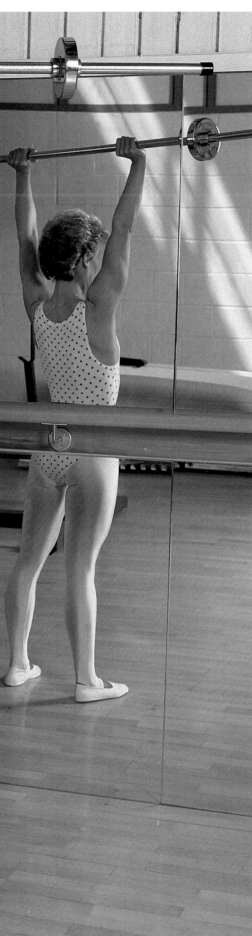

The press

Having cleaned the bar off the floor, and with the elbows well up, and without any body movement, press the bar overhead without looking at it, passing it as close as possible to your face on its upward journey. Reach up as far as possible but do not raise the heels off the floor (center). Brace the thighs and buttocks before commencing the press. Lower the weight back to the starting position and repeat. Use only the back and shoulder muscles and do not lean back in any way.
Breathing: Inhale just as you commence the press; exhale as you return to the starting position.

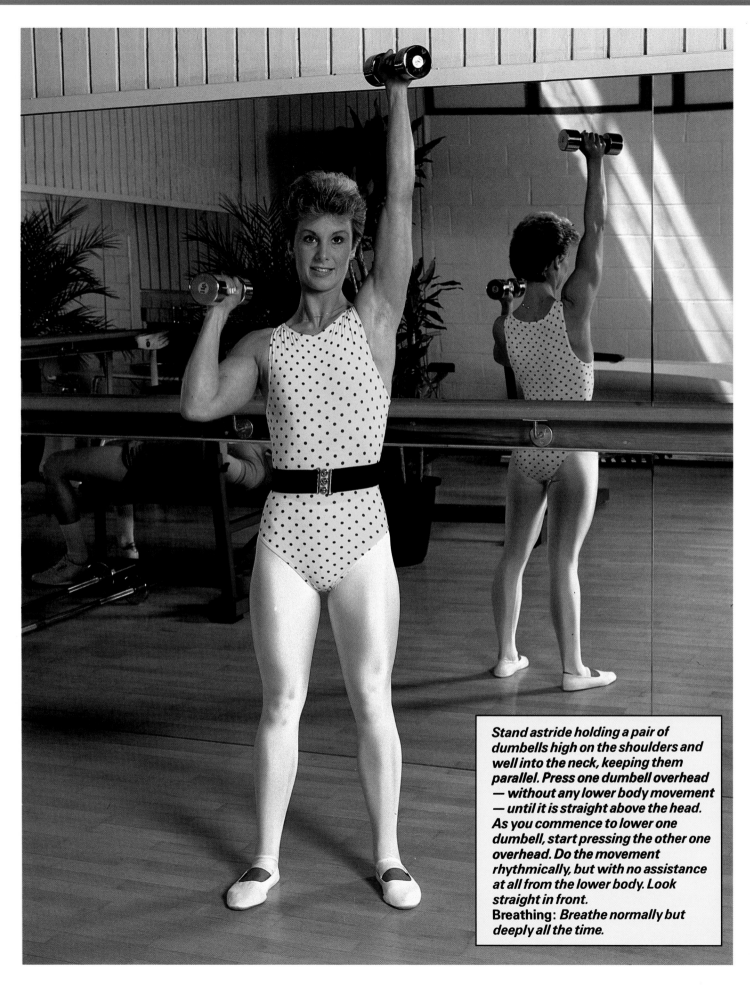

Stand astride holding a pair of dumbells high on the shoulders and well into the neck, keeping them parallel. Press one dumbell overhead — without any lower body movement — until it is straight above the head. As you commence to lower one dumbell, start pressing the other one overhead. Do the movement rhythmically, but with no assistance at all from the lower body. Look straight in front.

Breathing: Breathe normally but deeply all the time.

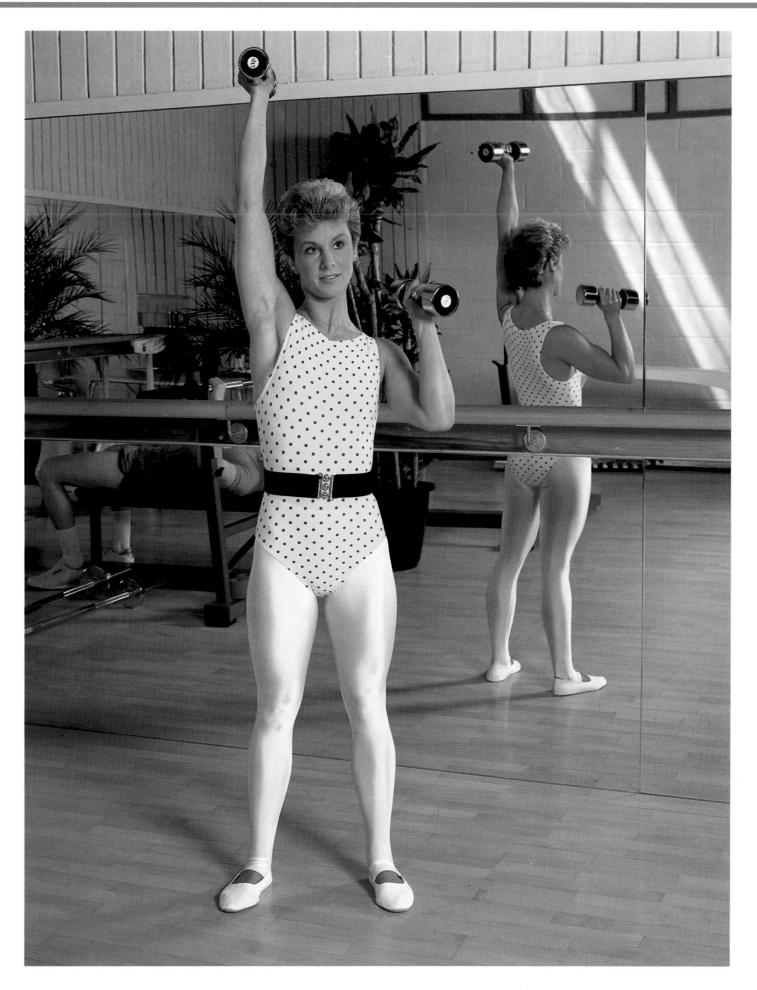

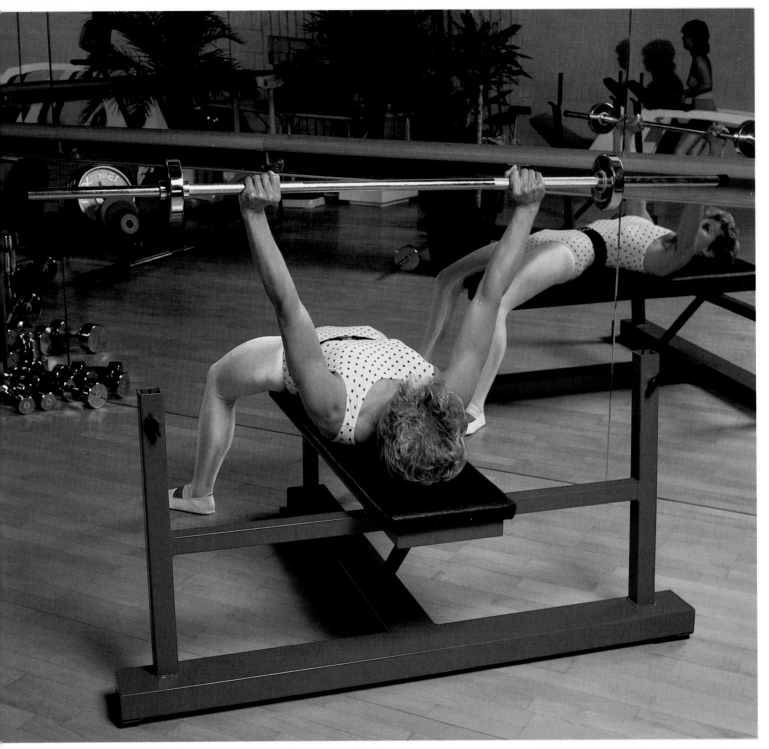

Lie on a bench, feet either side of it, and flat on the floor.
Get a training partner to hand you the barbell at arms' length above your head, even if there is a rack at the end of the bench.
Take a fairly wide grip, knuckles uppermost (above left). Lower the bar, keeping it fairly high until it touches the upper part of your chest (above right). Press the bar back to the overhead position and repeat.

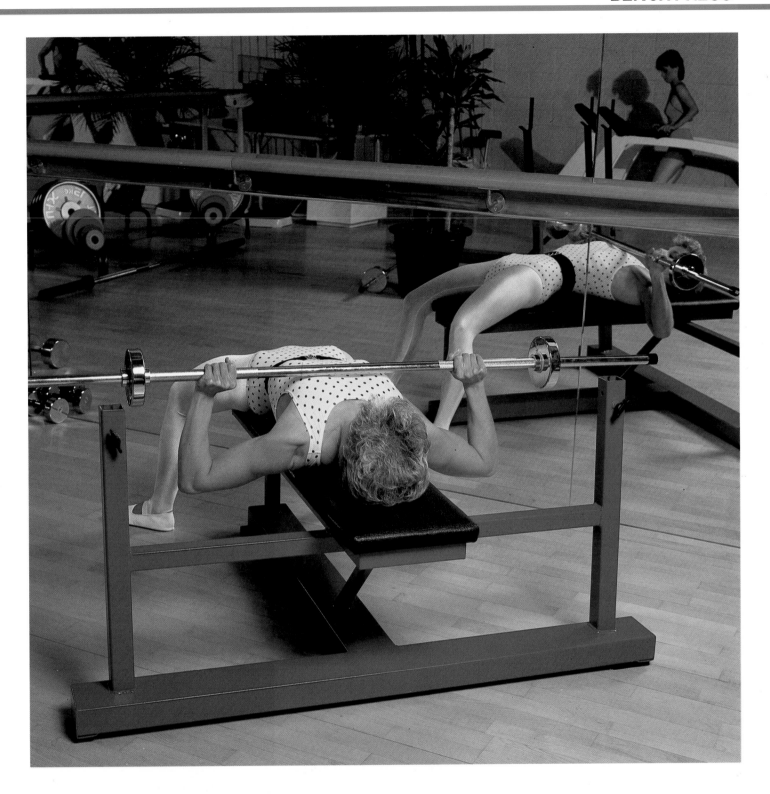

Breathing: *Inhale deeply as you lower the bar to the chest; exhale as you return it to the overhead position. This exercise strengthens the chest muscles and improves and firms the bust. It is also good for the arms, forearms and shoulders.*

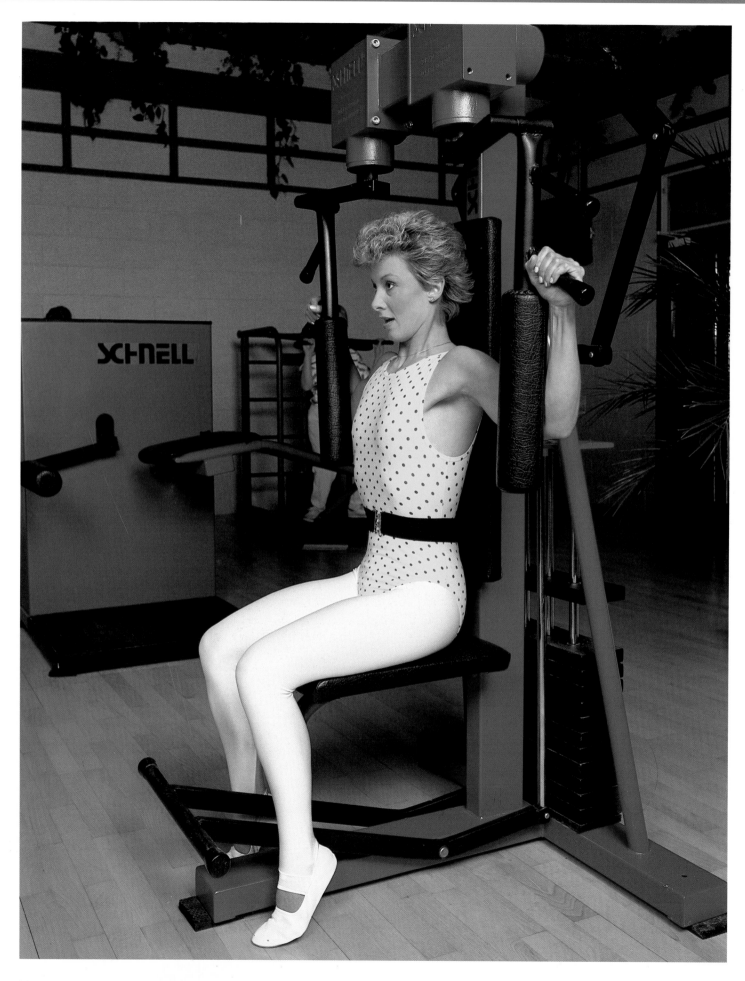

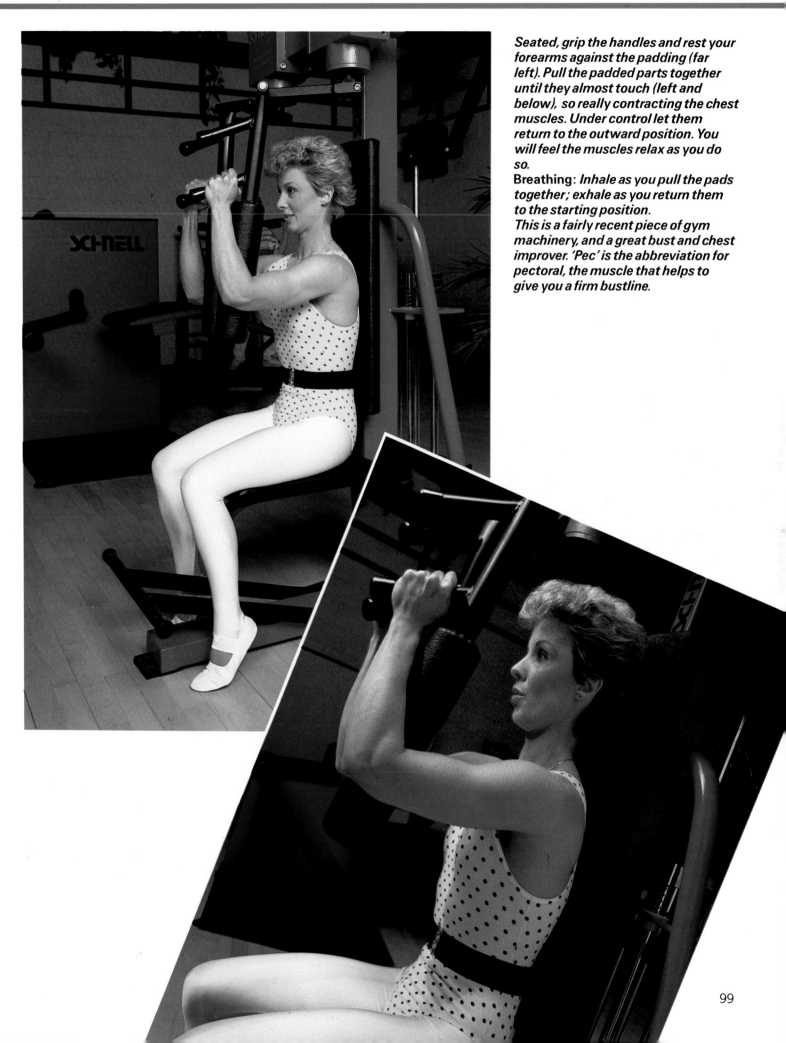

Seated, grip the handles and rest your forearms against the padding (far left). Pull the padded parts together until they almost touch (left and below), so really contracting the chest muscles. Under control let them return to the outward position. You will feel the muscles relax as you do so.

Breathing: *Inhale as you pull the pads together; exhale as you return them to the starting position.*

This is a fairly recent piece of gym machinery, and a great bust and chest improver. 'Pec' is the abbreviation for pectoral, the muscle that helps to give you a firm bustline.

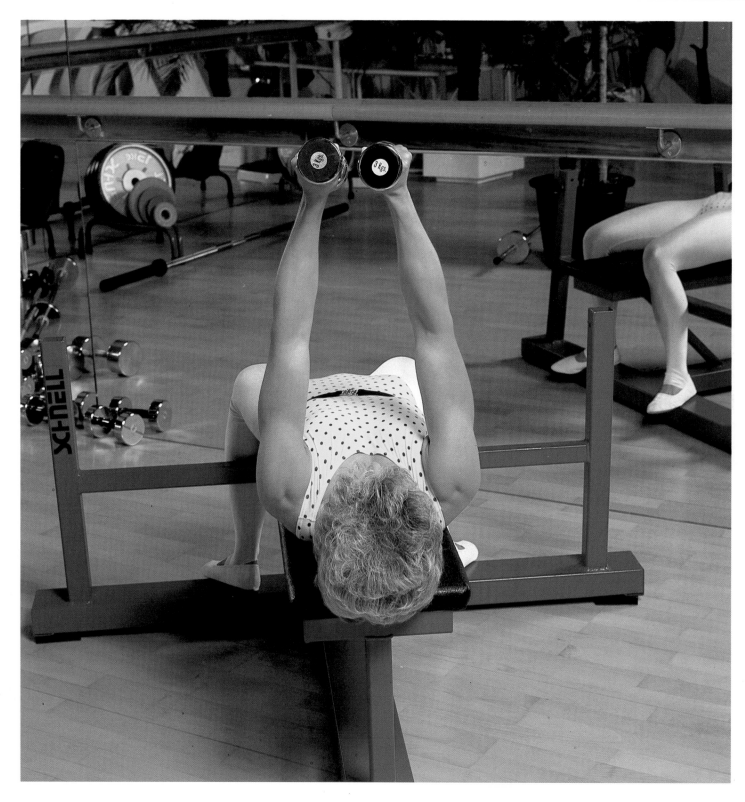

Lie on a bench with your feet on either side of it. Hold a pair of dumbells overhead, keeping them parallel and close together (above left). By bending the elbows, lower the dumbells outwards, but at first do not attempt to use too wide an angle, and never attempt to do this exercise with arms quite straight.

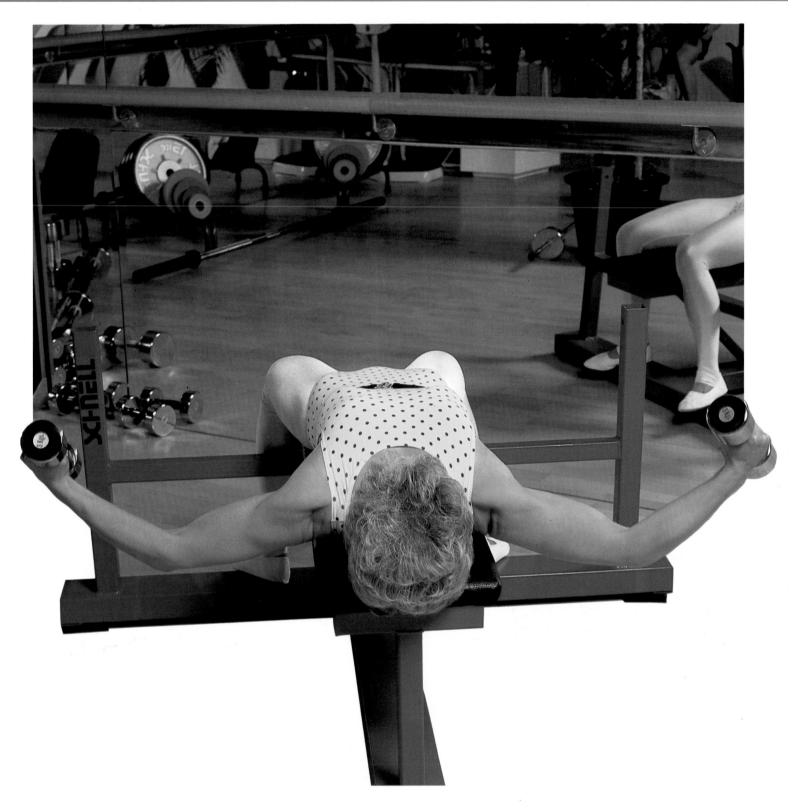

As soon as you have taken the dumbells as far as you can (above right), 'drag' them back to the starting position, feeling your chest muscles tense up.
Breathing: *Inhale as the dumbells go outwards; exhale as you return them overhead and parallel.*
A fine exercise for the bust and chest, and also good for the forearms.

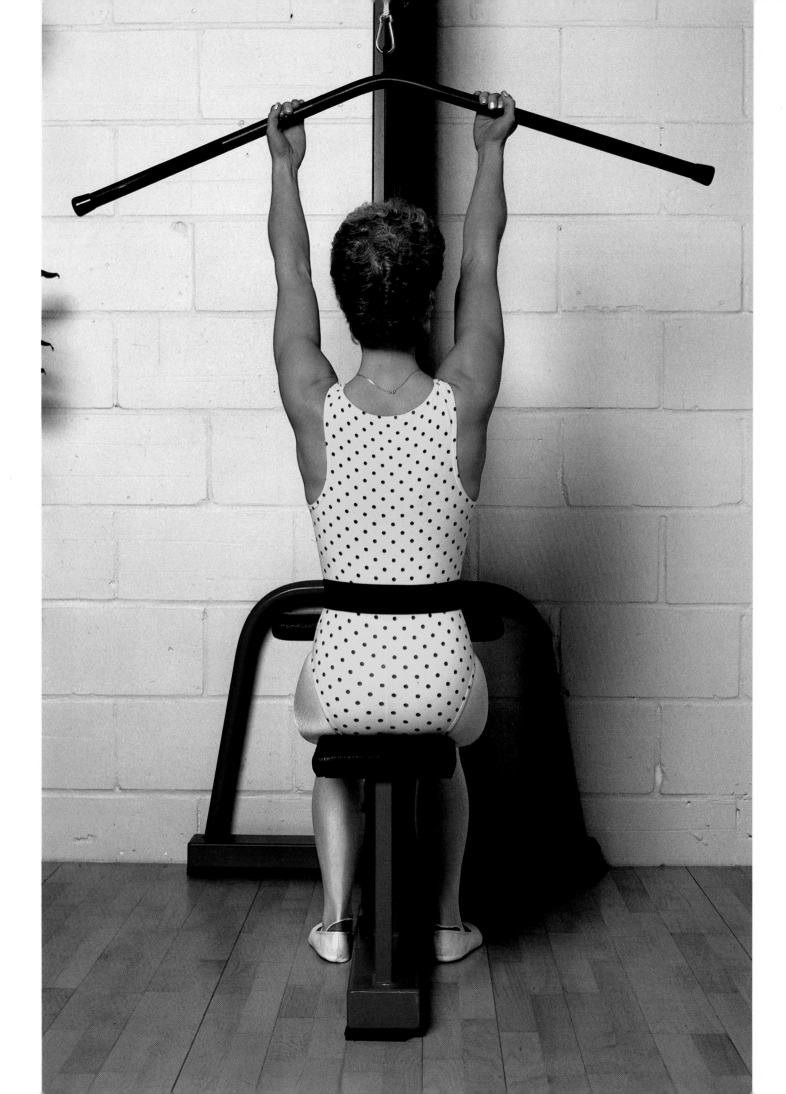

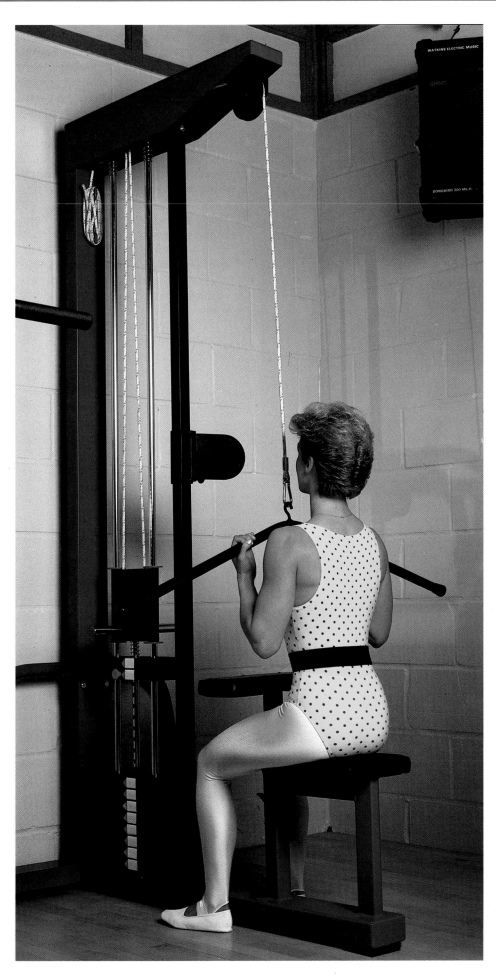

In this exercise you face the pulley and take a narrow grip (far left). Using the arms and chest muscles, pull the bar right down to the lower part of your chest keeping the elbows well into your sides (left).

It is quite a different exercise from the Pulley Pull to Back of Neck, and an excellent one for an older or less fit person.

Breathing: *Inhale deeply as you make the pull to chest; exhale as you return it to the starting position above the head.*

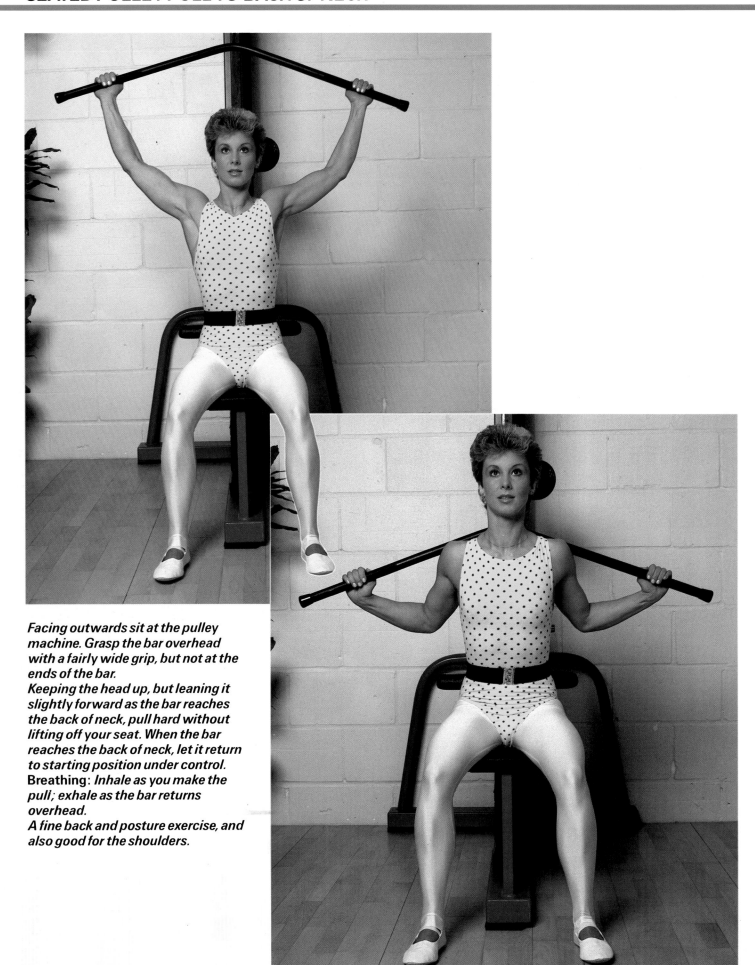

Facing outwards sit at the pulley machine. Grasp the bar overhead with a fairly wide grip, but not at the ends of the bar.

Keeping the head up, but leaning it slightly forward as the bar reaches the back of neck, pull hard without lifting off your seat. When the bar reaches the back of neck, let it return to starting position under control.

Breathing: *Inhale as you make the pull; exhale as the bar returns overhead.*

A fine back and posture exercise, and also good for the shoulders.

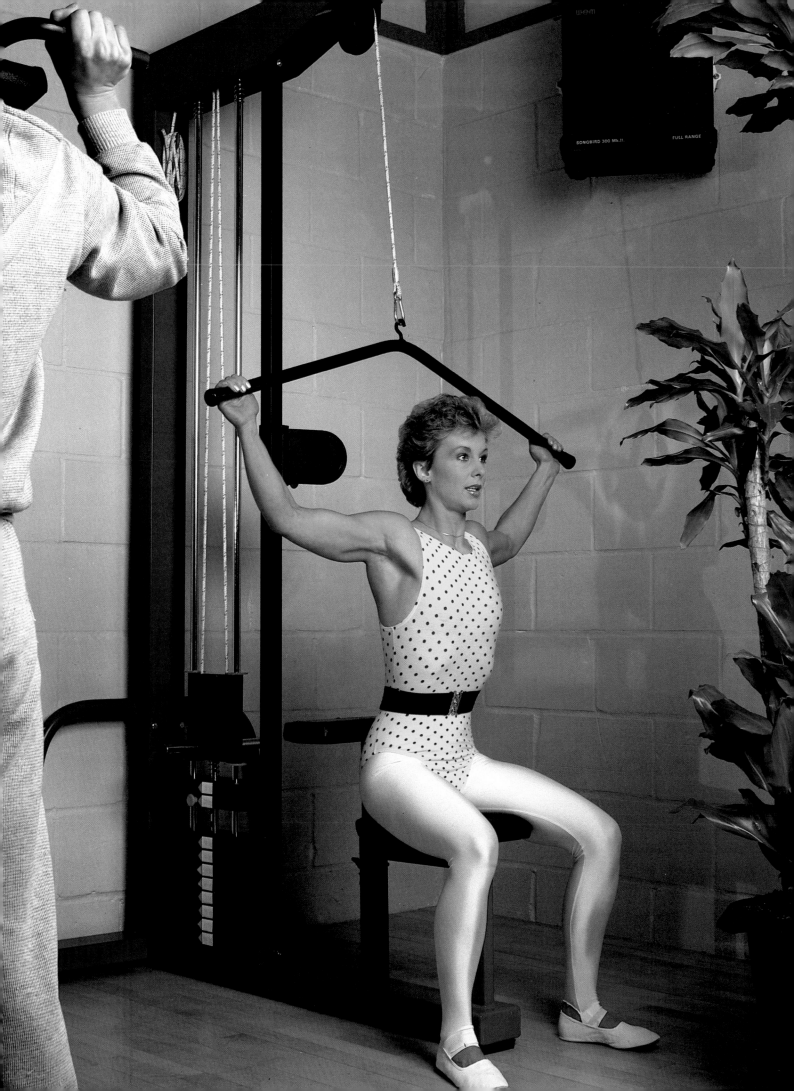

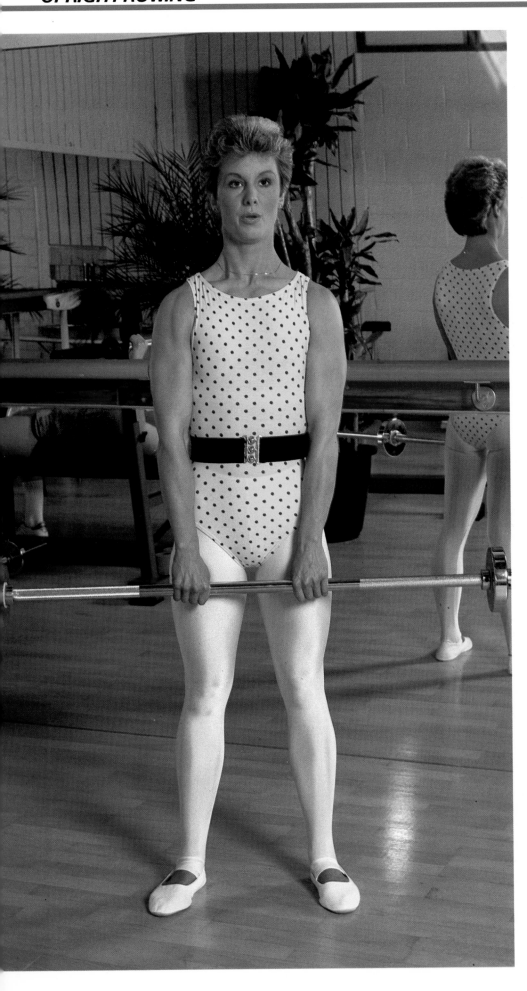

Stand astride holding a bar with a narrow grip, knuckles uppermost (left).
Pull the bar up towards the neck, by raising the elbows high (right).
Keep the bar always as near as possible to your body. The movement must come from the shoulders and chest. Do not move the legs at all.
Breathing: *Inhale as you pull the bar under the chin; exhale as you return it to in front of the hips.*

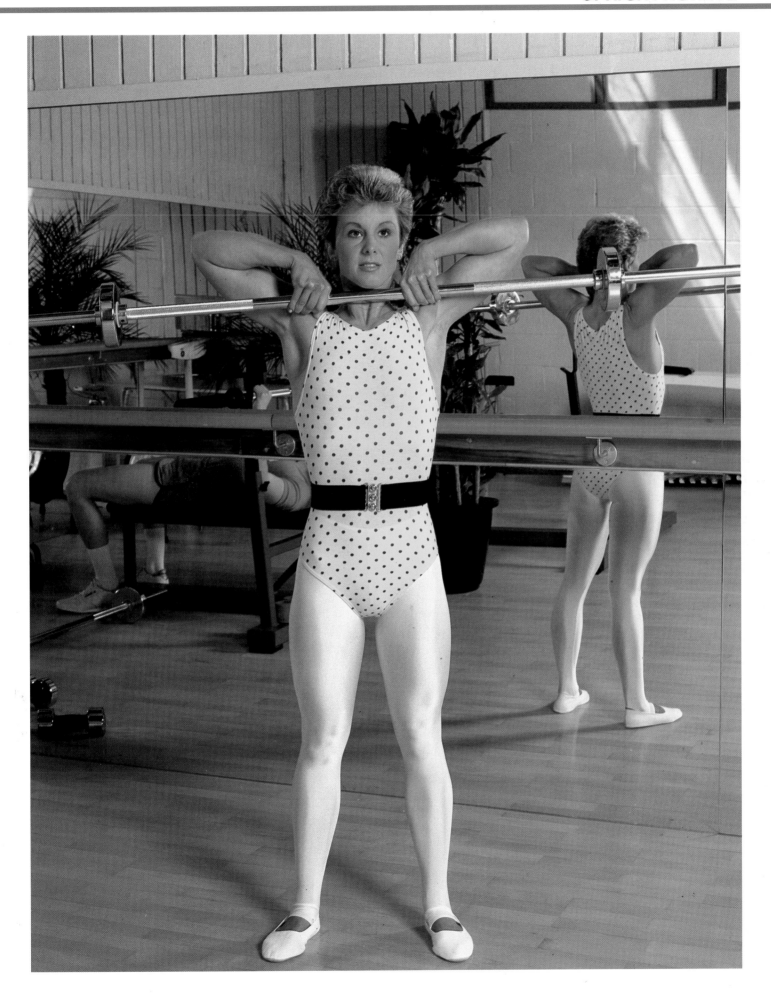

THE SQUAT (KNEES BEND)

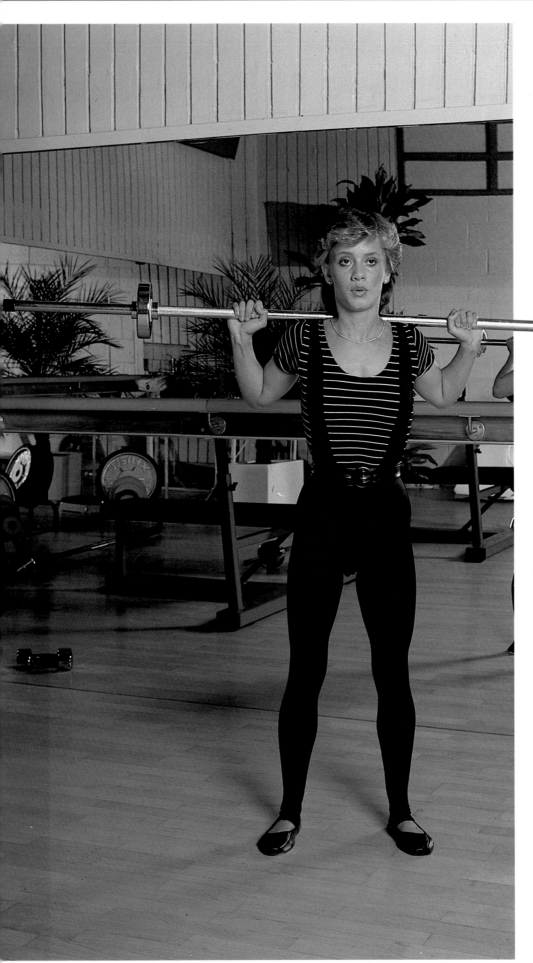

This is a great deal more than just a thigh and hip exercise. It is a must in almost any program for a younger and fairly fit woman. It is also used today by top sportspeople. A great power and endurance builder it has a marked affect on the respiratory system.

If you train at home and have no racks to support the barbell, have a training partner help you. Cover the back of your neck with a pad or the bar may mark your neck.

With the bar across your shoulders (left), take a deep breath, and leaning the body forward, but keeping your back perfectly straight (above right), bend the knees until the thighs are parallel with the floor (below right). As soon as your thighs are parallel to the floor, rise to starting position and repeat.

The toes must point to the front, and under no circumstances let your heels come off the floor. This in many cases is not easy, especially if you have been used to wearing high heels. Try without any weight and see if you can keep your feet flat on the floor.

If your heels rise off the floor, as they may well do, place a block of wood two or three inches high under your heels.

Breathing: Inhale deeply just as you start going down, and exhale as you are almost back at the starting position.

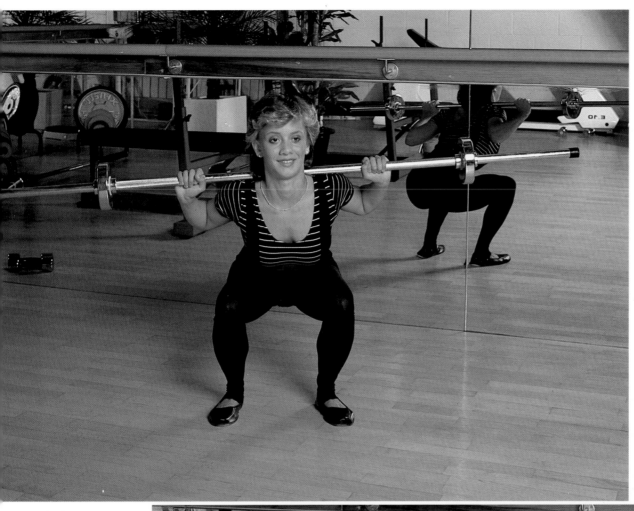

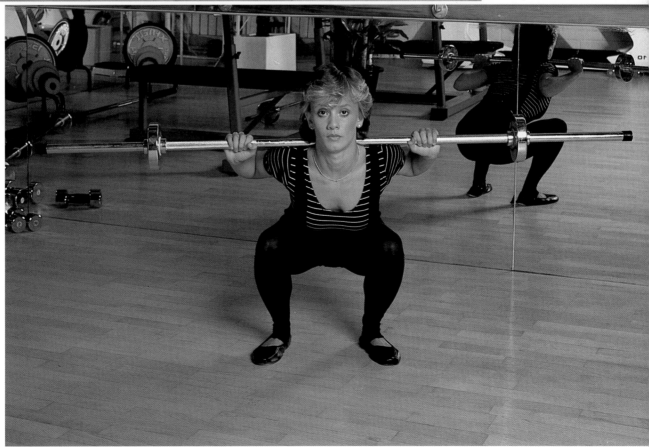

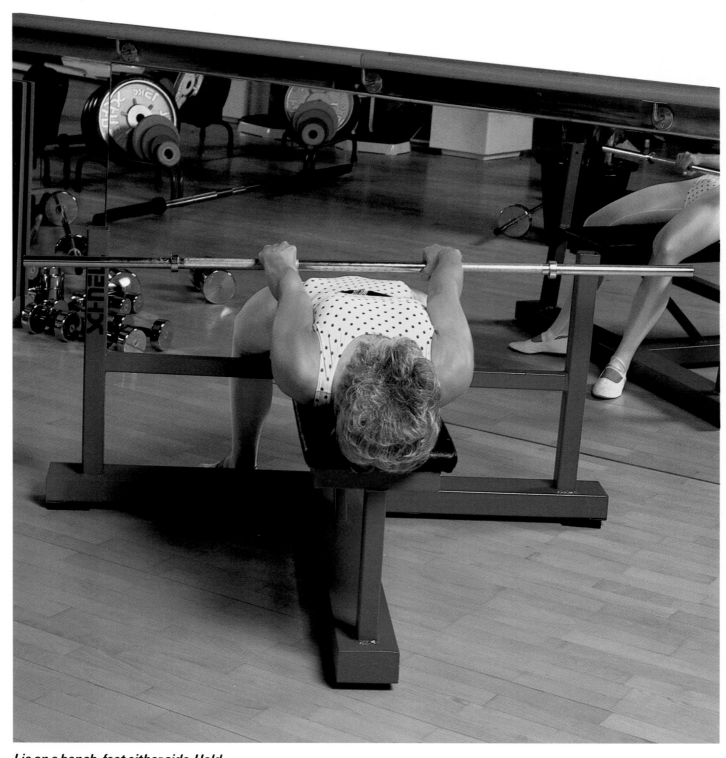

Lie on a bench, feet either side. Hold the bar at arms' length above the head. Keeping the elbows slightly bent, as it is a strong exercise, lower the bar with arms not altering until the bar is in line with the shoulders (above right). Pull the bar back to the overhead position above the head and lower it the other way to the thighs (above left). At first only do the beginning part of the exercise from the overhead position to behind with the arms in line with the body.

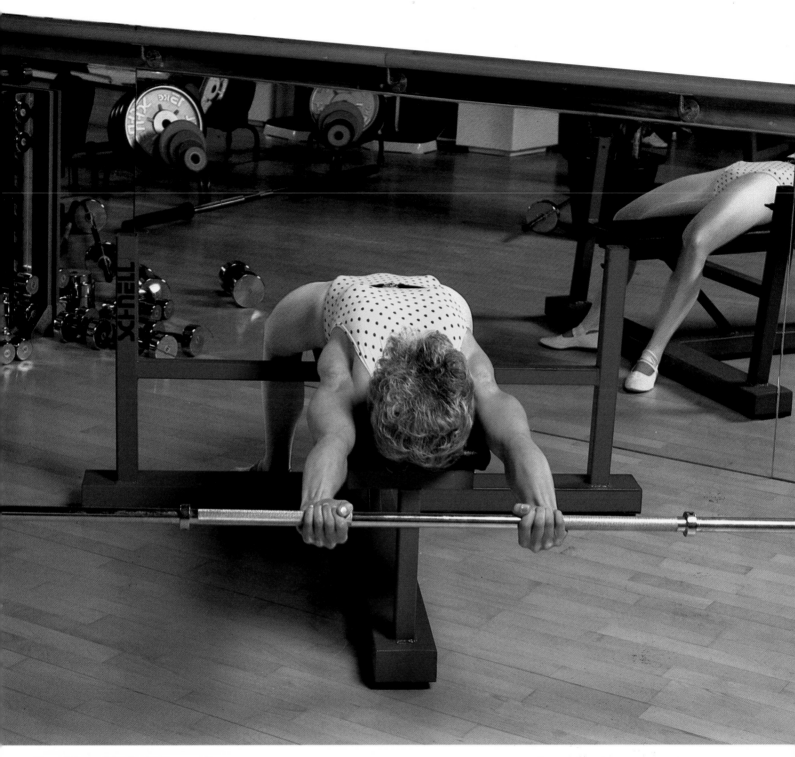

Breathing: *Inhale all the way from lowering the bar behind the head, and exhale as it touches the thighs. This is a great exercise for stretching the rib box and improving the posture. It also has a very marked effect on the respiration, and is usually done following the squat.*

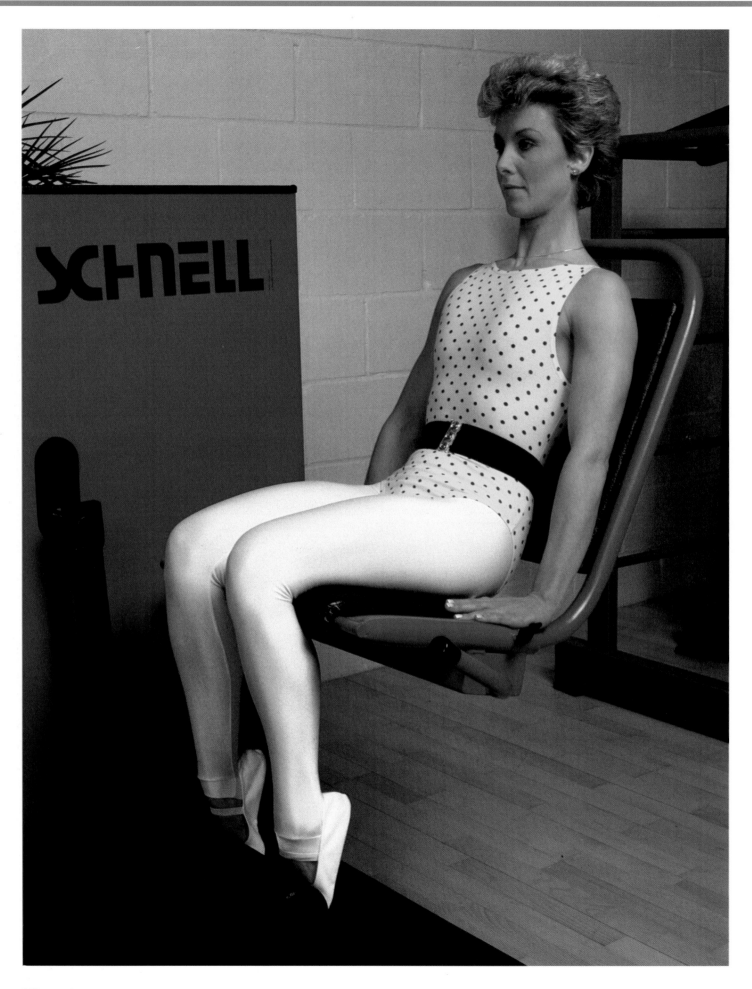

Sit at the extension machine, with the insteps under the bar, so that the legs are at right-angles to the body (left). Holding the side of the bench you are sitting on, extend the legs (right) until they are in a straight line in front of you (below). You will feel the thigh muscles contract; hold the position for a second or two and return to the starting position. Use a light weight and perform the exercise strictly.

Breathing: *Inhale as you make your effort; exhale as you lower the bar to the starting position.*

Leg extension machines are found in all modern health clubs. They are particularly good for strengthening the thigh muscles, and for those who have had minor knee problems. They are not as good as the squats, but do isolate the big muscles of the thighs more, and make them firmer and more shapely.

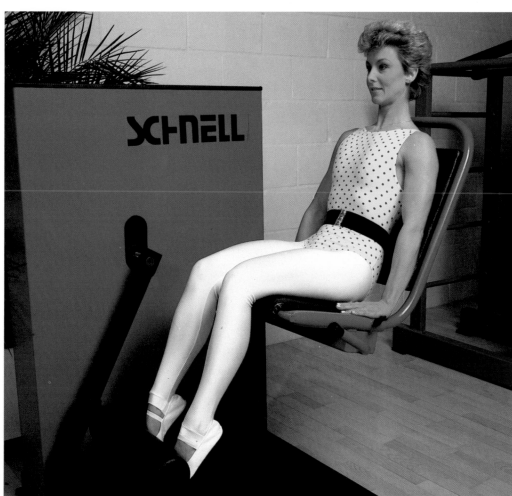

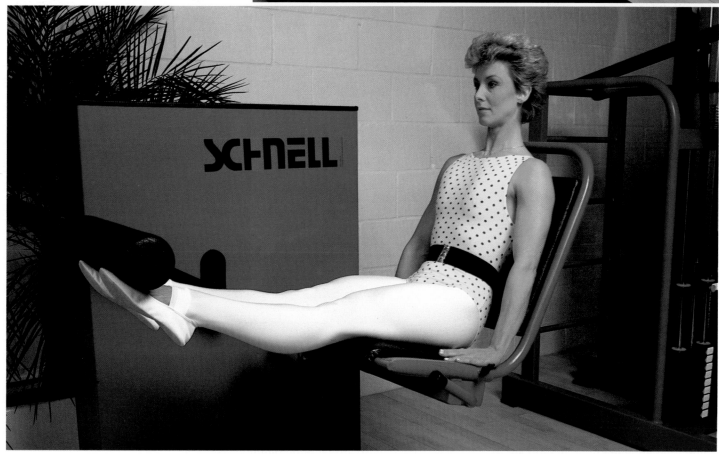

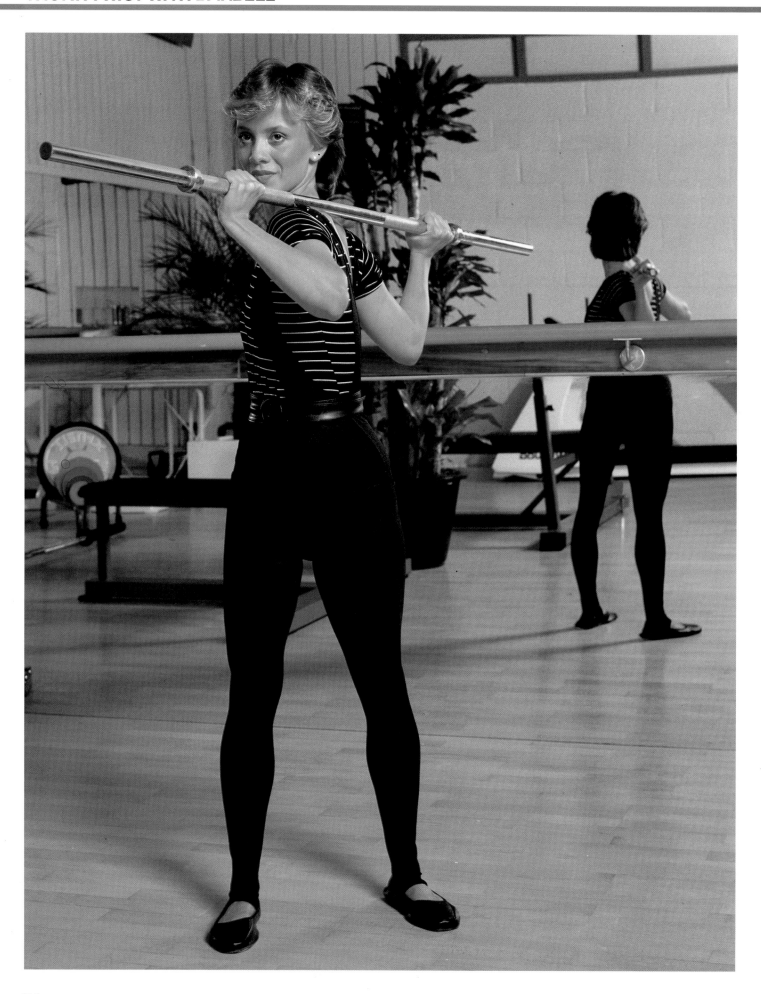

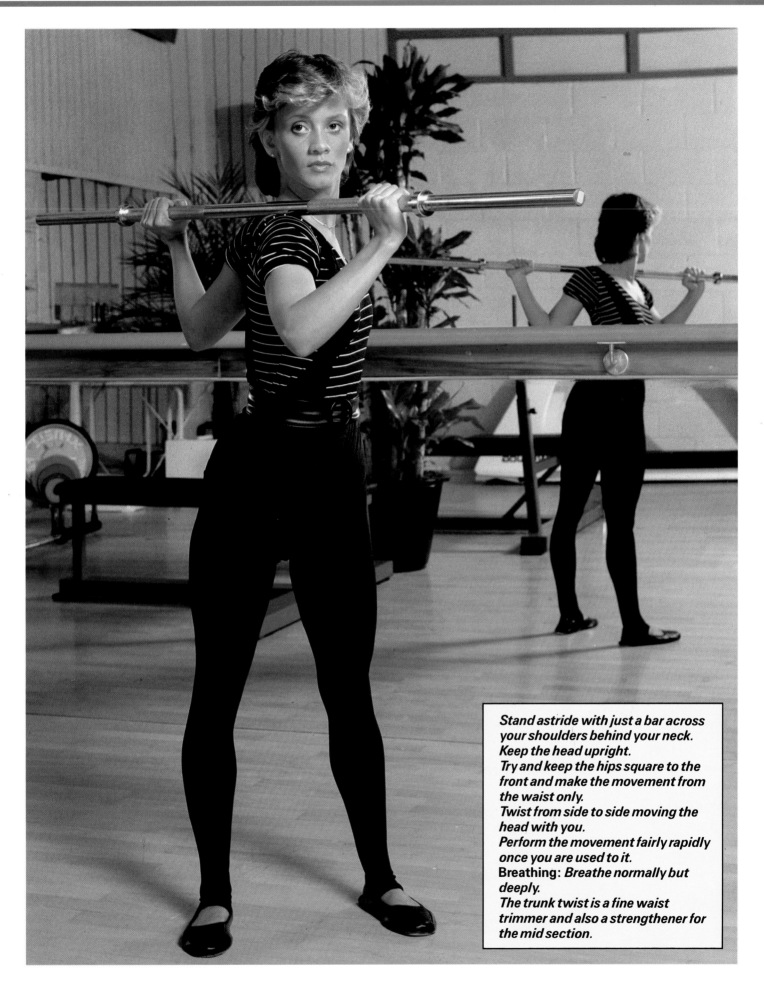

Stand astride with just a bar across your shoulders behind your neck. Keep the head upright.
Try and keep the hips square to the front and make the movement from the waist only.
Twist from side to side moving the head with you.
Perform the movement fairly rapidly once you are used to it.
Breathing: *Breathe normally but deeply.*
The trunk twist is a fine waist trimmer and also a strengthener for the mid section.

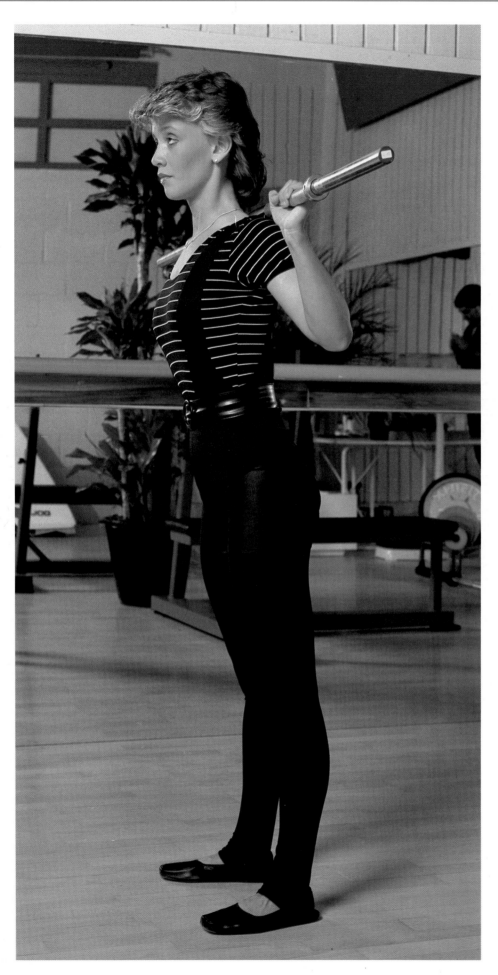

This is in your freestanding program, but to make the exercise a bit stronger, try it with a light barbell across your shoulders.

Stand feet astride with the bar behind your neck. Moving only from the waist, bend from side to side in a rhythm, but ensure that your body stays square to the front and that the muscles at the sides do the work. This is where your 'spare tire' is usually located so here is a chance to help get rid of it.

Breathing: *Breathe normally and let your head bend sideways with the bar.*

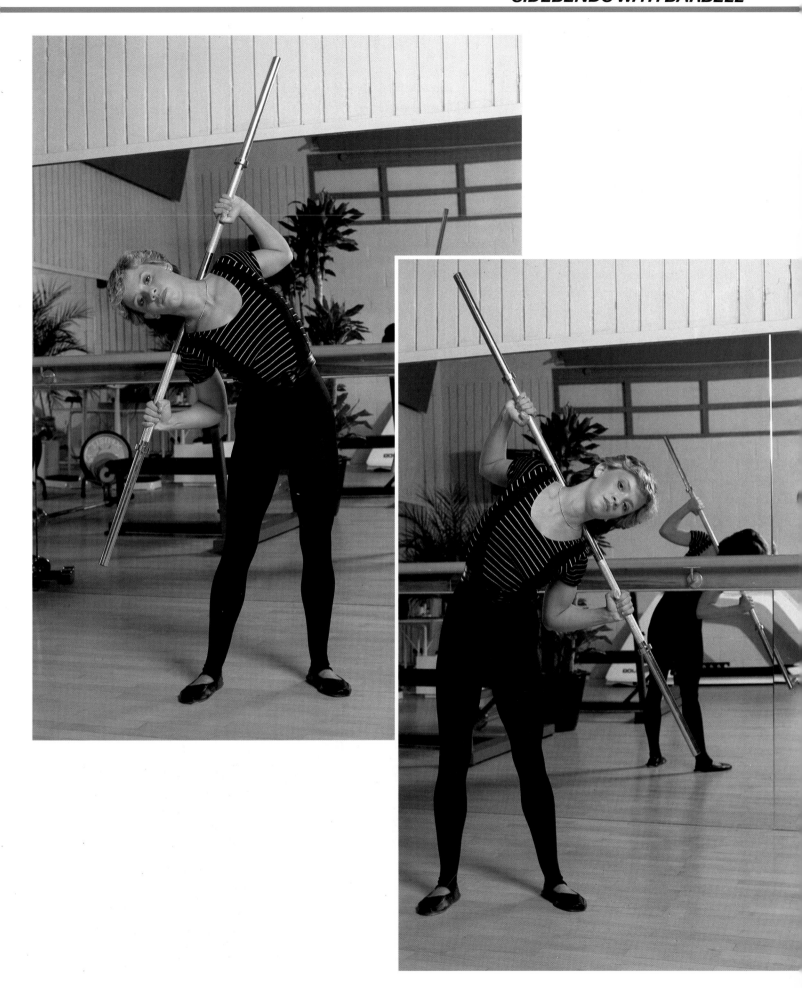

This may not seem very important, but it is. Never rush from your last exercise straight to the sauna or shower. Or stand and have a chin wag.

Lie on the floor after every workout for about three minutes. Knees raised, feet flat on the floor. Knees need not be pressed together but must be relaxed.

Arms at sides, palms of hands on floor. Close your eyes and try to imagine you are taking all the natural curves out of your spine and flattening it against the floor.

Breathing: Breathe slowly and deeply, in and out, until you feel you cannot take in any more air, and until you feel that you have exhaled completely.

Relaxation is intended mainly to return your respiratory system and heart and pulse rate to normal after the strain of the exercise program.

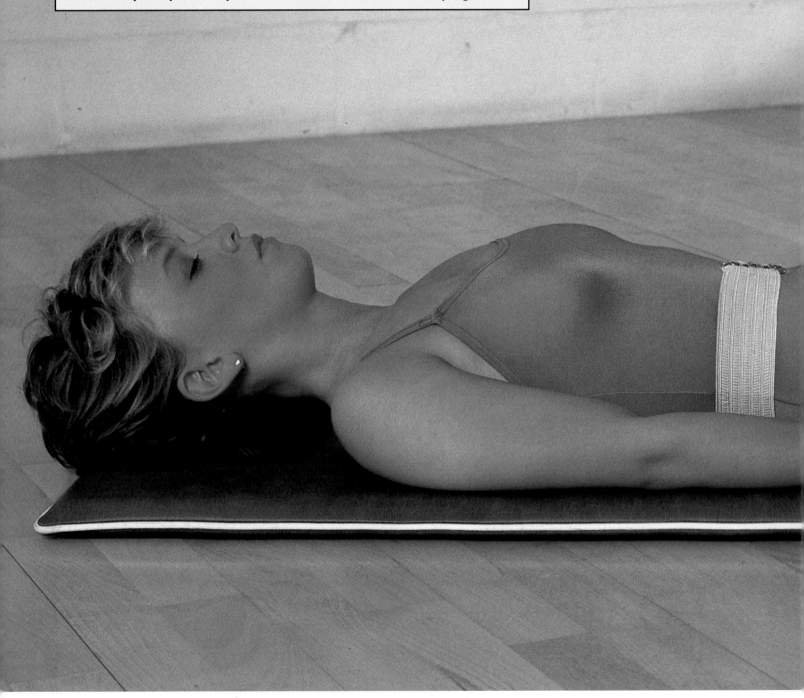

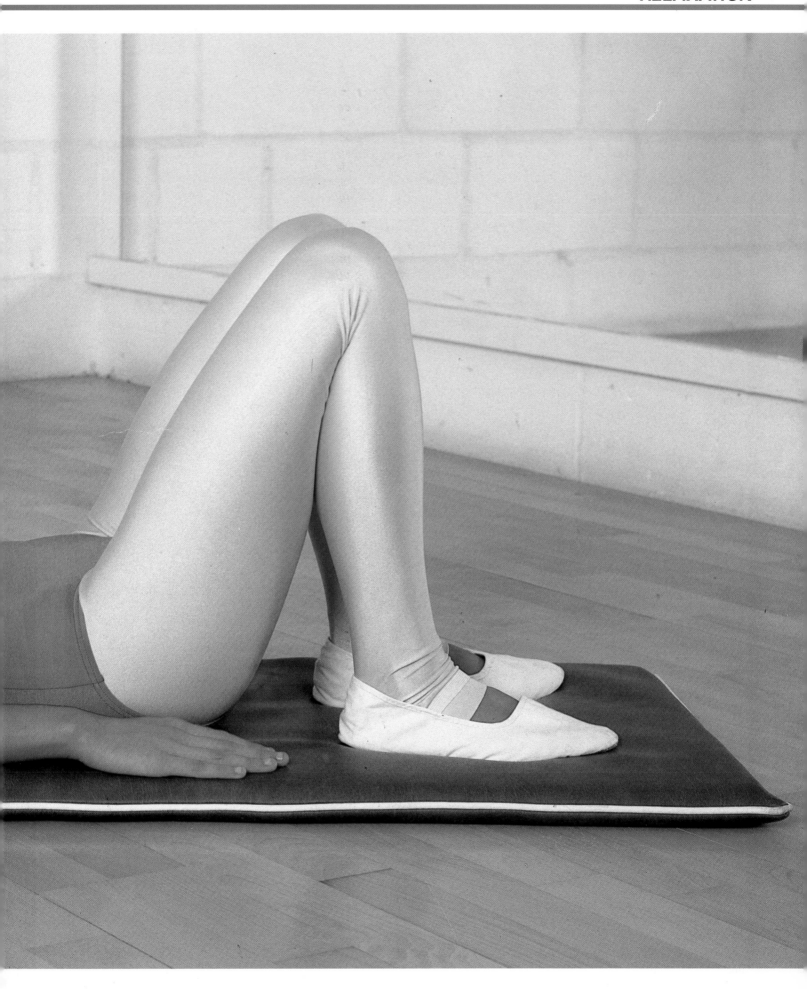

PICTURE CREDITS

120

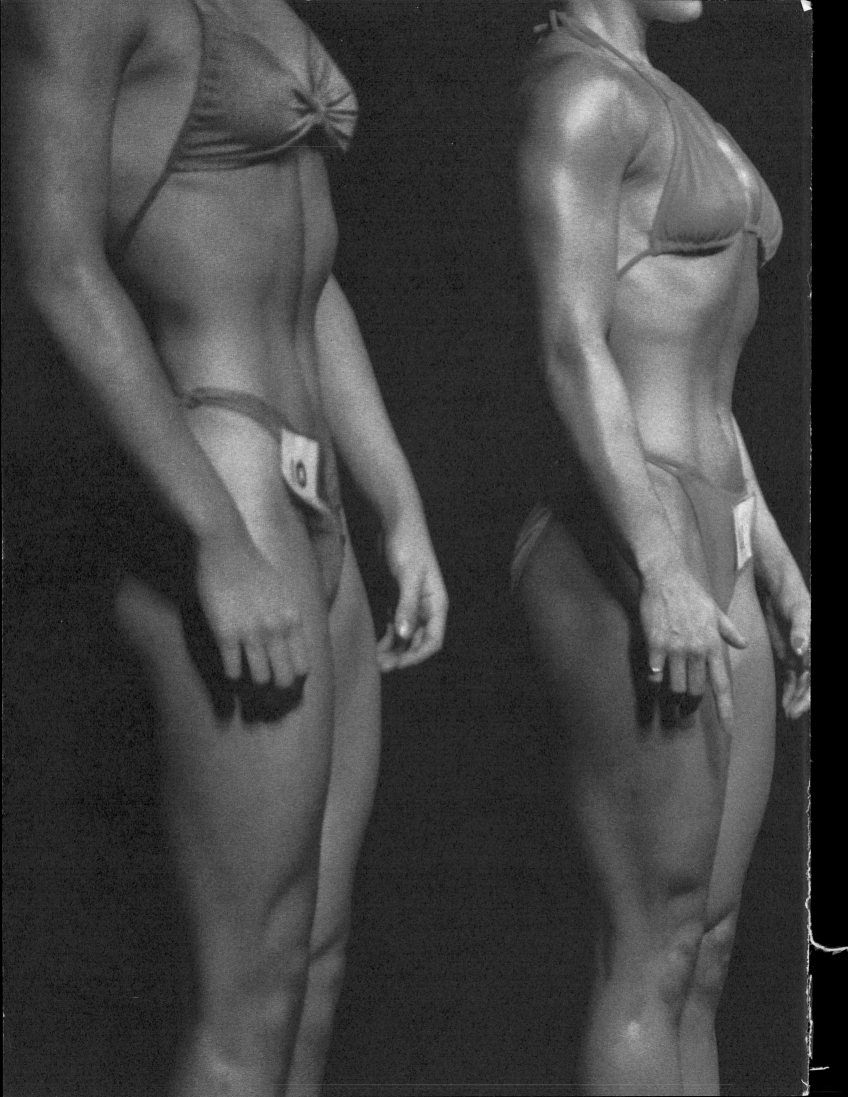